Practice MCQs for the final FRCA

Jonathan G Hardman
Lecturer
University Department of Anaesthesia
University Hospital
Nottingham

Ravi P Mahajan
Senior Lecturer (Honorary Consultant)
University Department of Anaesthesia
University Hospital
Nottingham

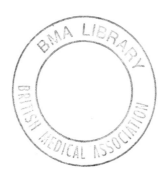

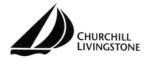

CHURCHILL
LIVINGSTONE

EDINBURGH LONDON NEW YORK PHILADELPHIA ST LOUIS SYDNEY TORONTO 1999

CHURCHILL LIVINGSTONE
An imprint of Harcourt Publishers Limited

First published 1999

ISBN 0 443 05311 1

British Library Cataloguing in Publication Data
A catalogue record for this book is available from the
British Library

Library of Congress Cataloging in Publication Data
A catalog record for this book is available from the
Library of Congress

Note
Medical knowledge is constantly changing. As new
information becomes available, changes in treatment,
procedures, equipment and the use of drugs become
necessary. The authors and the publishers have, as far
as it is possible, taken care to ensure that the information
given in this text is accurate and up to date. However,
readers are strongly advised to confirm that the
information, especially with regard to drug usage,
complies with the latest legislation and standards of
practice.

The
publisher's
policy is to use
paper manufactured
from sustainable forests

Printed in China

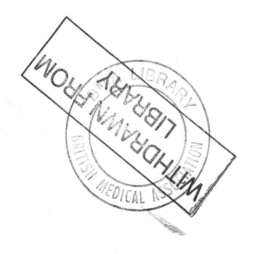

Commissioning Editor: Mike Parkinson
Project Editors: Sarah Keer-Keer & Jane Shanks
Project Controller: Frances Affleck
Designer: Erik Bigland

Preface

This book is intended to assist those preparing for the Royal College of Anaesthetists' final fellowship examination. The subject matter of the multiple-choice questions is based closely upon the syllabus published by the Royal College of Anaesthetists. It is hoped that this book may also be useful to those studying for other parts of the fellowship examination and for those preparing for anaesthesia examinations in other parts of the world.

The book is split into 10 exams: each contains 40 questions, with each question having five sections. Each section is answered as true or false, or you may abstain from answering. Each paper may be used as a practice examination, or the subject index can be used to allow the candidate to dip into the book following revision of a particular topic. The subject index is arranged by topics taken from the examination syllabus and lists all the questions dealing with each topic. In the spirit of the examination itself, each question may cover several topics.

In preparing this book, we have consulted the following reference texts: *Anesthesia and Co-existing Disease* (3rd edition), Stoelting; *Anesthesia* (4th edition), Miller; *Textbook of Anaesthesia* (3rd edition), Aitkenhead and Smith; *Clinical Anaesthesia* (1st edition), Aitkenhead and Jones; and *Clinical Medicine* (3rd edition), Kumar and Clarke.

We hope that readers enjoy this book and find it a useful aid to preparation for their examination. We wish you the best of luck in your endeavours.

JGH & RPM, 1999

Contents

Paper 1

1   **Regarding chronic medication and surgery under general anaesthesia:**
   A Angiotensin-converting enzyme inhibitors may potentiate hypertensive responses to intubation.
   B Withdrawal of short-acting antihypertensives is more dangerous than withdrawal of long-acting agents.
   C Antihypertensive agents may cause an increased risk of awareness.
   D Antihypertensives may reduce anaesthetic requirements.
   E Calcium channel blockers may potentiate bradycardia, negative inotropism and vasodilatation under general anaesthesia.

2   **In rheumatoid arthritis:**
   A Radiological cervical involvement is a feature in approximately 86% of cases.
   B Voice changes indicate possible cricoarytenoid involvement.
   C Significant renal impairment is as common in seronegative as in seropositive disease.
   D Respiratory function tests feature an obstructive or restrictive picture.
   E Cervical flexion is typically more dangerous than extension in rheumatoid cervical instability.

3   **Regarding the asthmatic patient presenting for surgery:**
   A Anticholinergic premedication is useful as a drying agent and bronchodilator.
   B Thoracic epidural analgesia causes problems because of intercostal paralysis and bronchoconstriction due to thoracic sympathetic blockade.
   C Anticholinesterase drugs given to reverse neuromuscular blockers may precipitate bronchospasm.
   D Mechanical ventilation should incorporate a prolonged inspiratory time.
   E Sodium cromoglycate may be used acutely to treat atopic asthmatic attacks.

Answers

---

1   A **False**   They may cause hypotension.
     B **False**   Rebound effects are more likely with withdrawal of
                    long-acting agents.
     C **True**   β-blockers may mask the signs of awareness.
     D **True** α_2-blockers may reduce anaesthetic requirements.
     E **True**

2   A **True**
     B **True**   The temporomandibular joint may also be involved,
                    causing difficulty in airway management.
     C **False**   It is only common in seropositive disease.
     D **True**   Bony deformity causes a restrictive picture, while
                    small airway involvement causes obstruction.
     E **True**   Flexion causes the odontoid peg to impinge upon
                    the cervical cord.

3   A **False**   Drying of secretions may cause worsening of the
                    asthmatic.
     B **False**   This is not a practical problem. The analgesia
                    afforded by epidural analgesia protects against
                    hypoventilation following abdominal and thoracic
                    surgery.
     C **True**
     D **False**   A long expiratory time should be used.
     E **False**   Cromoglycate is useful prophylaxis against atopic
                    bronchospasm, but has no role in acute
                    management.

4   **Concerning β-blockers:**

A They are competitive antagonists.
B The antihypertensive action is mediated via the kidneys.
C Heart failure is less likely with β_1-selective agents.
D β-blockers with intrinsic sympathomimetic activity are agonist–antagonists.
E They increase the risk of left ventricular end-diastolic pressure.

5   **Regarding the non-steroidal anti-inflammatory drugs (NSAIDs):**

A NSAIDs have an antipyretic action by inhibiting the formation of prostaglandin E_2.
B NSAIDs reduce the gastric secretion of mucus.
C Platelet aggregation is impaired by NSAIDs owing to the inhibition of thromboxane E_2 production.
D NSAIDs commonly cause bronchospasm in known asthmatics.
E High-dose aspirin is a recognised treatment for pregnancy-induced hypertension.

6   **Regarding non-invasive methods of cardiac output measurement:**

A Cardiac output may be measured by placing a Doppler ultrasound probe in the suprasternal notch, the oesophagus or the trachea.
B When measuring cardiac output with an ultrasound probe, a nomogram of great vessel cross-sectional areas may be necessary.
C Impedance plethysmography is inaccurate when pulse pressure is widened.
D Cardiac output measurement using transoesophageal Doppler can reasonably detect a change of 5%.
E Impedance plethysmography is of comparable accuracy to invasive methods.

7   **Regarding the monitoring of neuromuscular block:**

A Double-burst stimulation lasts less than 1 s.
B Double-burst stimulation is more accurate but more difficult to detect manually than train-of-four stimulation.
C The nerve stimulator should be able to produce a constant voltage for a variety of currents.
D Tetanic stimulation at 100 Hz or above may show tetanic fade in the absence of neuromuscular block.
E For accurate mechanomyography, a preload must be applied.

4   A   **True**
    B   **True**   It is also mediated via the heart and via presynaptic action in the brain.
    C   **False**
    D   **False**   They are weak partial agonists.
    E   **True**

5   A   **True**   This is mediated in the thalamus.
    B   **True**   This mucus protects the gastric mucosa.
    C   **False**   Thromboxane A_2 production is inhibited.
    D   **False**   Aspirin intolerance is seen in some asthmatics, often in the company of nasal polyps and chronic urticaria, but it is rare.
    E   **False**   Low-dose aspirin is gaining some favour. In doses of 50–150 mg.day^{-1} it is probably not a contraindication to epidural analgesia.

6   A   **True**
    B   **True**   Alternatively, the area may be measured with a suprasternal probe.
    C   **False**   It is less accurate when there is a loss of pulsatility.
    D   **False**   It can reasonably detect changes as small as 15%.
    E   **False**

7   A   **False**   It comprises two 0.2 ms stimuli separated by a 750 ms pause.
    B   **False**   It is easier to detect manually.
    C   **False**   It should be able to produce a constant current over a range of impedance.
    D   **True**   Presumably due to depletion of transmitter stores.
    E   **True**

8   Etomidate:

A   Is based upon a carbimazole ring.
B   Has a therapeutic index of approximately 26.
C   Is presented in 35% ethylene glycol.
D   Commonly produces nausea and vomiting.
E   Blocks adrenal mitochondrial enzymes after a single induction dose.

9   Regarding the attainment of equilibrium during volatile anaesthesia:

A   Volatile agent metabolism reduces the time constant for equilibration.
B   Halothane metabolism is a first-order process throughout the clinically useful range of doses.
C   During administration of a constant concentration of a volatile agent the blood tension is always lower than alveolar tension.
D   Trichloroethylene is heavily metabolised and has active metabolites.
E   The total body uptake of volatile agents may be easily measured using a servo-controlled closed circuit.

10   During bowel surgery:

A   Morphine increases the rate of anastomotic breakdown.
B   The use of neostigmine should be avoided.
C   Atropine is more effective than glycopyrrolate in inhibiting the gastrointestinal effects of neostigmine.
D   Antibiotics may potentiate competitive muscle relaxants.
E   Perioperative changes in plasma cortisol levels are reduced by the use of extradural opioids.

11   Regarding open cholecystectomy:

A   Kocher's incision is considerably more painful than an upper right paramedian incision.
B   Any opioid may induce spasm in the sphincter of Oddi.
C   Spasm in the sphincter of Oddi may be reversed with naloxone.
D   Patients are often obese.
E   Kocher's incision is amenable to analgesia via intercostal blocks or psoas compartment blocks.

8 A **False** It is based upon an imidazole ring.
   B **True**   It is thus very safe in terms of immediate effects.
   C **False** It is presented in 35% propylene glycol.
   D **True**   30% of adults receiving etomidate will suffer nausea and vomiting.
   E **True**   The reduction in cortisol and aldosterone production lasts for at least 24 h.

9 A **False** It increases it.
   B **False** Halothane metabolism is saturated at 2–10% of MAC, making it then a zero-order process.
   C **True**   Metabolism and loss through the skin account for the difference.
   D **True**   The active metabolite is trichloroethanol.
   E **True**   This is the easiest way.

10 A **False** This has not been demonstrated despite several studies.
   B **True**   This dramatically increases bowel activity, possibly risking anastomotic breakdown.
   C **True**
   D **True**   Aminoglycosides can do this.
   E **True**   The stress response is diminished.

11 A **True**   It is not used as often these days because of the associated pain.
   B **False** Opioids with pure agonist action may induce spasm.
   C **True**   This demonstrates that the action is related to action on opioid receptors.
   D **True**   This is associated with the formation of gallstones.
   E **False** Paravertebral, intercostal or epidural blockade is useful. Psoas compartment blocks are too low.

12   A pulmonary artery flotation catheter yields the following data: cardiac index 2.07 l.min^{-1}.m^{-2}, systemic vascular resistance index 3001 dyn.s.cm^{-5}.m^2, pulmonary capillary wedge pressure 20.2 mmHg and central venous pressure 2.8 mmHg.

A   Mean arterial pressure is 70 mmHg.
B   One cannot state whether the vascular resistance is normal without knowing the height and weight of the patient.
C   This patient would probably benefit from rapid infusion of fluids.
D   Pulmonary capillary wedge pressure is usually slightly higher than pulmonary arterial diastolic pressure and thus more accurately represents left atrial pressure.
E   Systemic vascular resistance is greater in large patients than in small patients.

13   Regarding independent lung ventilation:

A   It requires two ventilators.
B   It should only be used if both lungs have similar compliance.
C   It should be synchronised so that both lungs are inflated at the same time.
D   It is more safely administered using a bronchial blocker than a double-lumen endobronchial tube.
E   Greater positive end-expiratory pressure should be applied to the lung with larger compliance.

14   Regarding calcium metabolism:

A   Most calcium absorption takes place in the duodenum by active transport.
B   Calcitriol is produced in the kidney under the influence of parathyroid hormone.
C   Calcitonin increases bone resorption.
D   Parathyroid hormone increases plasma calcium and plasma phosphate levels.
E   99% of body calcium is found in bone.

15   Regarding peritoneal lavage following trauma:

A   It may be safer than abdominal computed tomography.
B   It is both sensitive and specific for intra-abdominal bleeding.
C   It is preferable to abdominal ultrasound during resuscitation of an adult.
D   Access to the peritoneum is usually gained above the umbilicus.
E   200 ml of warmed saline should be introduced into the abdomen.

12	A	**False**	(MAP – CVP) = CI × SVRI/80. Mean arterial pressure is thus approximately 80 mmHg.
	B	**False**	SVRI is independent of size. SVRI = SVR × BSA.
	C	**False**	This patient probably has left ventricular failure and would benefit from diuretics and possibly inotropes.
	D	False	Backward flow is almost never seen in the PA, so PCWP is usually lower than PADP.
	E	**False**	SVR falls as patient size increases. SVRI is independent of patient size.

13	A	**True**	
	B	**False**	One of the commonest reasons for using it is a disparity in the compliance of the two lungs.
	C	**False**	This is unnecessary.
	D	**False**	A bronchial blocker will prevent ventilation of one of the lungs.
	E	**False**	The lung with the lower compliance will have a smaller FRC and greater shunting. PEEP will be most beneficial here.

14	A	**True**	It is regulated by 1,25-dihydroxycholecalciferol.
	B	**True**	
	C	**False**	It reduces bone resorption, reducing serum calcium and phosphate levels.
	D	**False**	It increases ionised plasma calcium levels and reduces plasma phosphate levels.
	E	**True**	

15	A	**True**	Transfer to the (often remote) CT suite is dangerous in traumatised patients.
	B	**False**	It is not very specific, since it may cause bleeding itself. It is, however, cheap and quick.
	C	**True**	
	D	**False**	It should be gained below the umbilicus.
	E	**False**	One litre of warm saline should be used. 200 ml may not drain.

16   Positive end-expiratory pressure:

A Increases FRC.
B Reduces alveolar deadspace.
C Markedly increases atrial natriuretic peptide secretion.
D Increases CVP.
E Reduces PCWP.

17   Pancuronium:

A Is sympatholytic.
B Is one of the more anaphylactogenic muscle relaxants.
C Is a quaternary amine.
D Is not used in obstetric practice since it readily crosses the placenta.
E Is used in cardiac anaesthesia because of its minimal cardiovascular side effects.

18   Thiopentone:

A Is a methylbarbiturate.
B Initially undergoes first-order kinetics in large doses.
C Is proconvulsant in large doses.
D May be mixed with muscle relaxants.
E Is analgesic even at sub-anaesthetic doses.

19   Regarding the cardiac action potential:

A Ca^{2+} channels are not important in the pacemaker areas.
B Phase 0 of the action potential represents rapid influx of sodium ions into the myocyte.
C Cardiac muscle is relaxed during the refractory period.
D Phase 4 slow depolarisation is due to slow K^+ efflux.
E Resting membrane potential is increased by increased extracellular K^+ concentration.

20   The following will affect the measurement of mean arterial pressure:

A Height of the transducer.
B Compliance of the tubing.
C Length of the tubing.
D Resonance within the transduction system.
E Inclusion of an air bubble within the tubing.

16 A **True**   This is the basis of its beneficial effect.
    B **False**
    C **False**   Extrinsic compression of the atria may reduce ANP
                  secretion.
    D **True**   Right ventricular afterload is increased.
    E **True**   This is due to the rise in PVR.

17 A **False**   It is sympathomimetic.
    B **False**   It is relatively rarely associated with anaphylactic
                  reactions.
    C **True**   It is thus almost entirely ionised in vivo and does not
                  cross the blood–brain barrier, renal tubule or the
                  placenta.
    D **False**   See above.
    E **False**   It is used in cardiac anaesthesia because of its mild
                  sympathomimetic effects.

18 A **False**   It is a thiobarbiturate.
    B **False**   In large doses it undergoes zero-order kinetics.
                  When plasma levels fall significantly, its metabolism
                  may switch to first order, as the liver enzymes are no
                  longer saturated.
    C **False**   It is anticonvulsant.
    D **False**   It forms an insoluble precipitate when mixed with
                  acidic solutions.
    E **False**   It may be anti-analgesic – increasing the patient's
                  sensitivity to pain.

19 A **False**
    B **True**
    C **False**
    D **True**
    E **True**

20 A **True**   Pressure is measured at the height of the transducer
                  and compared with the zero point. Elevation of the
                  transducer will lower the apparent arterial pressure.
    B **False**   Compliant tubing causes damping of the signal,
                  lowering systolic and elevating diastolic pressure
                  measurements. The mean pressure is unaffected.
    C **False**   Adding length to the tubing has the same effect as
                  increasing the compliance of the tubing.
    D **False**   This has the opposite effect as damping. Mean
                  pressure is unaffected, while pulse pressure is
                  increased.
    E **False**   This causes damping of the signal.

21   The following may influence the accuracy of indirect blood pressure determination:

A Size of blood pressure cuff.
B Size of the bladder.
C Position of the bladder.
D Accuracy of the aneroid manometers.
E Site of measurement.

22   Drugs useful in the therapy of paroxysmal atrial tachycardia during operation include:

A Digoxin.
B Verapamil.
C Esmolol.
D Amiodarone.
E Quinidine.

23   The following factors do not have a significant effect on the duration and intensity of subarachnoid block:

A Baricity.
B Vasoconstrictors.
C Removal of drug by vascular absorption.
D Concentration of local anaesthetic.
E Addition of a spinal narcotic.

24   Regarding postdural puncture headache:

A It is more common in the elderly.
B It is not affected by the needle bevel direction.
C Needle tip design has an insignificant effect.
D It gets worse on lying prone.
E It is mainly occipital and not frontal.

21 A **True**
    B **True**
    C **True**
    D **True**
    E **True**
    All of the choices are correct. A cuff that is too wide relative to the circumference of the arm will give erroneously low pressures, and one that is too narrow will give incorrectly high estimates. The bladder should cover at least half of the circumference of the limb.

22 A **True**
    B **True**
    C **True**
    D **True**
    E **False**
    Other manoeuvres include carotid massage. Electrical cardioversion may be necessary.

23 A **False**
    B **False**
    C **False**
    D **False**
    E **False**
    Other factors that may affect the distribution and, therefore, duration and intensity of subarachnoid block may include the position of the patient during injection, dose of local anaesthetic and site of injection. Minor factors include age, height, volume of CSF, direction of the spinal needle and the anatomical configuration of the spine.

24 A **False**
    B **False**
    C **False**
    D **False**
    E **False**
    Postdural puncture headache is more common in younger patients and is affected by the design of the needle tip. Whittaker needles are found to be better than others. The direction of the needle bevel has some effect. Bevels cutting dural fibres longitudinally produce fewer headaches than those that cut the fibres transversely. The headache may get better lying prone, but certainly gets worse in a sitting posture. The headache can be bifrontal as well as occipital. It usually radiates to the neck and the shoulders.

25   Regarding ionised calcium:

A It has a positive inotropic effect.
B The effect of adrenaline on the myocardium is dependent on its availability.
C Its administration during CPR improves outcome only after the heart starts beating.
D It has limited value in clinical electromechanical dissociation.
E It is an important determinant of myocardial function in the intensive care unit.

26   A male patient of 60 years of age with long-standing hypertension well controlled on β-blockers is scheduled for inguinal hernia repair. He is otherwise well.

A He should not be operated upon in a day-case unit.
B He requires a very heavy premedication before surgery.
C He has the same risk for developing cardiac complications in the perioperative period as his normotensive counterpart.
D He is not a suitable candidate for regional anaesthesia.
E He should take his β-blocker a day before but not on the morning of surgery.

27   The following mechanisms are involved in inhibition of pain at the dorsal horn:

A Hyperpolarisation of nerve terminals mediated by opioid receptors.
B Hyperpolarisation of nerve terminals mediated by GABA receptors.
C α_2 stimulation.
D Descending inhibitory neurones releasing noradrenaline.
E Descending inhibitory neurones releasing 5-HT.

28   The following features are commonly seen in association with sepsis:

A Oliguria and renal failure despite increased cardiac output.
B The cardiovascular system is very sensitive to the effect of vasoactive agents.
C ARDS.
D Altered mental function.
E Respiratory acidosis at the onset of sepsis.

29   Common causes of postoperative hypotension include:

A Inadequate fluid replacement.
B Decreased myocardial contractility.
C Residual effect of anaesthetic drugs.
D Pain.
E Stress response.

25   A **True**
      B **True**
      C **False**   There is no such evidence.
      D **True**
      E **True**
Although calcium is essential for adequate cardiac muscular
activity in a variety of conditions, during CPR the main
indications are hyperkalaemia, hypocalcaemia or calcium
channel blocker overdose.

26   A **False**   He is ASA class 2.
      B **False**   Not necessary.
      C **False**   Risk is higher than in a normotensive patient.
      D **False**
      E **False**   Antihypertensive medication should be continued
                     until the morning of surgery.

27   A **True**
      B **True**
      C **True**
      D **True**
      E **True**
At the dorsal root level inhibitory neurotransmitters include
GABA, acetylcholine, α_2 agonists, opioids and serotonin. These
are released in response to signals from descending pathways
from higher centres.

28   A **True**
      B **False**   This system is more likely to be resistant to
                     vasoactive agents.
      C **True**
      D **True**
      E **False**   Minute ventilation increases owing to the
                     hypermetabolic state and hypoxia and this is more
                     likely to cause respiratory alkalosis.

29   A **True**
      B **True**
      C **True**
      D **False**   Hypertension is more likely in pain.
      E **False**

30   The following measures are recommended in the immediate management of venous air embolism:

A Aspiration of air using a pulmonary artery catheter.
B Irrigation of the site of operation.
C Placing the patient in right lateral position.
D Administration of vasodilators to reduce pulmonary vascular resistance.
E Thiopentone for cerebral protection.

31   Autonomic hyperreflexia following spinal cord transection:

A Is unlikely to be associated with injuries belowT10.
B Is usually manifested by hypertension and tachycardia.
C Results from loss of inhibitory control from higher centres.
D Can lead to cerebral haemorrhage.
E Results in vasodilatation above the level of injury.

32   The following are normal for a neonate:

A The oxyhaemoglobin dissociation curve is shifted to right to improve oxygen delivery.
B The effect of changes in the oxyhaemoglobin dissociation curve on oxygen delivery to tissues is offset to some extent by increased haematocrit.
C The prothrombin time is increased but the bleeding time is normal.
D Airway resistance is higher and the lung compliance is lower than in adults.
E The spinal cord ends at the lower border of L3.

33   Trisomy 21 (Down's syndrome) is associated with:

A Mental retardation.
B A high incidence of congenital heart disease.
C Airway abnormalities.
D Cervical spine instability.
E Increased incidence of postoperative pulmonary complications.

34   In a hypertrophied left ventricle associated with aortic stenosis:

A There is no role of atrial systole in assisting diastolic filling.
B Diastolic filling is unaffected.
C Ejection time is prolong ed.
D Pulmonary arterial occlusion pressure overestimates LVEDP.
E Ventricular compliance remains unaffected until the onset of heart failure.

30   A **True**
      B **True**
      C **False**   Left lateral position. This places the right side of the
                      heart upwards.
      D **False**
      E **False**
Immediate measures include 100% oxygen, flood the operation
site with saline, aspirate air from right side of heart and
inotropes to maintain blood pressure. If the problems persist
and the patient remains hypotensive with poor cardiac output
due to raised pulmonary vascular resistance, pulmonary
vasodilators and cerebral protection may be considered.

31   A **True**   Incidence is highest at levels above T6.
      B **False**   Hypertension and bradycardia are usual.
      C **True**
      D **True**
      E **True**   This may be diagnostic.

32   A **False**   Presence of HbF causes its shift to left.
      B **True**
      C **True**   There is deficiency of vitamin K dependent factors
                      but the blood coagulates probably because of
                      deficiency of naturally occurring anticoagulants.
      D **True**
      E **True**

33   A **True**
      B **True**
      C **True**
      D **True**
      E **True**

34   A **False**   Atrial systole contributes up to 30% of diastolic filling.
      B **False**   It is reduced due to decreased compliance of the
                      ventricle.
      C **True**   This further reduces the time available for diastolic
                      filling.
      D **False**   It actually underestimates LVEDP.
      E **False**   Heart failure is a late complication. Compliance is
                      affected very early in the disease process.

35   In pulmonary oedema subsequent to left ventricular failure:

A PCWP is likely to be 20 mmHg.
B Morphine helps by reducing the preload.
C Frusemide is effective only when it results in increased diuresis.
D Vasodilators are contraindicated.
E X-ray changes lag behind left atrial pressure changes.

36   Propranolol:

A Reduces plasma renin activity.
B Has intrinsic sympathomimetic activity.
C Is a selective blocker of β_2 receptors.
D Attenuates tachycardia induced by vasodilators.
E Unlike β_1 selective blockers has no effect on bronchial smooth muscles.

37   Hypertension following carotid endartectomy can be the result of:

A Denervation of carotid sinus.
B Pain.
C Full bladder.
D Hypoxia and hypercarbia.
E Trauma to the phrenic nerve.

38   Hepatorenal syndrome has the following characteristic features which differentiate it from acute tubular necrosis (ATN):

A Association with cirrhosis, ascites and portal hypertension.
B Poorer response to diuretics.
C Higher concentration of sodium in urine.
D Casts in urine.
E Higher urine/plasma creatinine ratio.

39   Immediate management after reperfusion of the transplanted liver should include:

A Fluids and blood to allow CVP between 10 and 15 mmHg in order to maintain adequate cardiac output.
B Nitroglycerine if the transplanted liver is congested.
C Sodium bicarbonate.
D Calcium chloride.
E Dobutamine.

35 A **False**   It is likely to be more than 30 mmHg.
    B **True**   Morphine is a known vasodilator.
    C **False**   The immediate action of frusemide is to decrease
                   preload by venular dilatation.
    D **False**   Vasodilators are used in treatment of left ventricular
                   failure to reduce preload as well as afterload.
    E **True**

36 A **True**
    B **False**
    C **False**   Blocks both β_1 as well as β_2 receptors.
    D **True**
    E **False** β_2 blockade due to propranolol can exacerbate
                   bronchospasm. β_1 selective blockers have
                   insignificant effects on bronchial smooth muscle.

37 A **True**   Denervation of the carotid sinus interferes with the
                   reflex control of increased blood pressure.
    B **True**
    C **True**
    D **True**
    E **False**   Phrenic nerve trauma can interfere with breathing
                   but not with blood pressure maintenance.

38 A **True**
    B **True**
    C **False**   Sodium is <10 mmol.l^{-1} compared to 50–70 mmol.l^{-1}
                   in ATN.
    D **False**   Characteristic feature of ATN.
    E **True**   In ATN urine/plasma creatinine is < 20.

39 A **False**   CVP should be maintained at the lower side of
                   normal to prevent congestion in the transplanted
                   liver.
    B **True**
    C **True**
    D **True**
    E **True**
Acidosis and low serum calcium are well known during
reperfusion. Dobutamine increases the cardiac output and
maintains splanchnic blood flow.

40   The following are recognised features in chronic renal failure:

A Malnutrition.
B Neuropathies.
C Susceptibility to infection.
D Gout.
E Myocardial dysfunction.

40   A **True**
     B **True**
     C **True**
     D **False**
     E **True**

Other risk features associated with renal disease are hypertension, cardiomegaly, anaemia, coagulation abnormalities, pleural effusions, biochemical abnormalities and acid–base upsets. Gout is not a typical feature of CRF, while renal dysfunction can result from hyperuricaemia in gout.

Paper 2

41 Regarding preoperative medication:

A Digitalised patients should receive atropine before induction to protect against bradyarrhythmias.

B Anticonvulsants should be withdrawn prior to surgery because of their unpredictable effects on anaesthesia.

C Benzodiazepines have no effect on the action of muscle relaxant drugs.

D In patients taking steroids, additional steroid cover is only required for major procedures.

E Preoperative administration of magnesium prolongs neuromuscular blockade.

42 Regarding preoperative investigations:

A 20% of chest X-rays demonstrate abnormalities.

B A positive Sickledex test should always be followed by serum electrophoresis.

C Blood chemistry analysis provides unexpected abnormal results in only 1% of patients under 40 years of age.

D Exercise stress testing is the most useful assessment of cardiac ventricular dysfunction.

E Coagulation studies may demonstrate abnormalities caused by chronic non-steroidal anti-inflammatory use.

43 Regarding cystic fibrosis:

A It usually leads to significant obesity.

B Bronchiectasis, cor pulmonale and chronic *Pseudomonas* infections are common.

C Blood gases often demonstrate hypoxaemia and hypocapnia.

D It usually results in death before the age of 14 years.

E Pancreatic insufficiency necessitates intravenous feeding after major procedures.

44 Regarding diuretic agents:

A Hypokalaemia and hyperkalaemia are seen.

B Thiazide diuretics increase calcium excretion.

C Loop diuretics cause hypomagnesaemia.

D Amiloride potentiates the effects of competitive muscle relaxants.

E The benefit of loop diuretics in pulmonary oedema is partly due to their diuretic action.

Answers

41 A **False**
    B **False**   Rebound effects may cause convulsions.
    C **False**   There is an additive effect with competitive
                   relaxants. Suxamethonium may be antagonised.
    D **False**   Additional steroid cover is required in the majority
                   of cases.
    E **True**

42 A **False**   Only 4% show any abnormality.
    B **True**   The patient may have HbS or HbSS.
    C **True**   This test is of little use in fit patients in this age
                   group.
    D **False**   Echocardiography is safe, non-invasive, sensitive
                   and specific.
    E **False**   Analysis of platelet function is necessary to detect
                   the effect of NSAIDs on clotting.

43 A **False**   Patients are usually underweight.
    B **True**
    C **False**   Patients are usually hypercapnic.
    D **False**   Life expectancy is around 20 years of age.
    E **False**   Oral pancreatic replacement is usually sufficient.

44 A **True**   Loop and thiazide diuretics cause hypokalaemia,
                   while potassium-sparing diuretics may cause
                   hyperkalaemia.
    B **False**   Loop diuretics increase calcium excretion, but
                   thiazides do not.
    C **True**
    D **False**   The potassium-losing diuretics (loop diuretics and
                   thiazides) can potentiate competitive relaxants.
    E **True**   They also acutely increase venous capacitance.

45   Regarding anticoagulant drugs:

A After oral administration, warfarin is bound to 97% of circulating albumin.

B Warfarin crosses the placenta freely, and is teratogenic in the first trimester.

C Vitamin K reverses the effect of warfarin, but makes the patient refractory to warfarin for up to 3 days.

D Heparin inhibits platelet function and increases the permeability of vessel walls.

E Low molecular weight heparin has a greater effect on thrombin than has mixed molecular weight heparin.

46   Regarding echocardiography:

A M-mode imaging scans in a fan-shaped pattern to give an anatomical display.

B During colour flow Doppler imaging, red, green and yellow code for blood speeds.

C The long-axis view during transoesophageal echocardiography visualises all chambers of the heart.

D Estimates of ejection fraction may be made from either long- or short-axis views during transoesophageal echocardiography.

E Afterload may be assessed using transoesophageal echocardiography.

47   Regarding hypothermia and the monitoring of body temperature:

A Hypothermia (<36°C) occurs in 30% of patients undergoing body cavity surgery.

B An ambient temperature of 21°C makes hypothermia unlikely in the adult undergoing surgery.

C Metabolic rate falls by 15% for each °C fall in body temperature.

D Tympanic temperature reflects hypothalamic temperature.

E A thermocouple's electrical resistance changes with temperature.

48   Regarding propofol:

A It is an isomethylphenol.

B It has a pK_a of 10.6.

C The vast majority is plasma protein bound.

D It causes pain on injection, which is moderated by pretreatment with fentanyl.

E It reduces the duration of fitting if given to provide anaesthesia for electroconvulsive therapy.

45 A **False**   97% of warfarin is bound to albumin, but much of the circulating albumin does not have warfarin bound to it.
    B **True**
    C **False**   The refractoriness may last for several weeks.
    D **True**   This increases the haemorrhagic effects of heparin.
    E **False**   Low molecular weight heparin has less effect on thrombin and more effect in catalysing the inhibition of factor Xa by antithrombin III.

46 A **False**   This is two-dimensional echocardiography.
    B **False**   Red and blue code for blood direction, while green codes for turbulent flow.
    C **True**
    D **True**
    E **True**   Calculation of end-systolic ventricular wall stress may be made by measurement of ventricular size, wall thickness and arterial pressure.

47 A **False**   It occurs in 75%.
    B **False**   Ambient temperature needs to be higher to prevent hypothermia.
    C **False**   It falls by 6–9% for each °C drop.
    D **True**
    E **False**   A thermistor's resistance changes with temperature. A thermocouple uses two dissimilar metals that develop a potential between them.

48 A **False**   It is an isopropylphenol.
    B **True**
    C **True**   97–98%.
    D **True**   Lignocaine is effective when mixed with the propofol. A large vein is less likely to hurt.
    E **True**   Although there is no evidence that it reduces efficacy of ECT.

49   Regarding the maintenance of volatile anaesthesia:

   A Halogenated volatile agents exhibit tachyphylaxis.
   B Patients may show acute tolerance to the analgesic effects of nitrous oxide.
   C Volatile agent requirement is higher in the chronic alcohol abuser.
   D Tolerance is often seen to halogenated volatile agents in patients undergoing repeated anaesthetics.
   E The central nervous response to volatile agents exhibits hysteresis in effect.

50   Regional anaesthesia for bowel surgery:

   A Is associated with less blood loss than general anaesthesia.
   B Increases the size of the postoperative negative nitrogen balance.
   C Requires a block extending from T6 to T12.
   D May make surgery more difficult because the bowel luminal diameter is reduced.
   E Reduces the cortisol response more than any general anaesthetic technique.

51   Regarding laparoscopic cholecystectomy:

   A It requires the insertion of a nasogastric tube.
   B It results in equal length of hospital stay when compared to open cholecystectomy.
   C Use of carbon dioxide as the inflating gas has been replaced by nitrogen since it interferes less with capnography.
   D Continuous flow of insufflation gas is required to compensate for that lost in expiration.
   E The head-down tilt required during gallbladder dissection may cause cardiovascular compromise.

52   The following data are collected from a 54-year-old man with a pulmonary artery flotation catheter in situ: mean pulmonary artery pressure 18.5 mmHg, pulmonary capillary wedge pressure 10 mmHg, pulmonary vascular resistance index 241 dyn.s.cm^{-5}.m^2, central venous pressure 2.7 mmHg, mean arterial pressure 48 mmHg.

   A His cardiac output is less than 50% of normal.
   B He is pathologically vasodilated.
   C He will benefit from rapid fluid infusion.
   D Infection is a likely cause of this situation.
   E Left ventricular stroke work index is likely to be elevated.

49 A **False**
    B **True**
    C **True**   This is probably due to tolerance.
    D **False**   This is not seen clinically. Experimental work with dogs also shows no tolerance.
    E **True**   Patients wake up with lower alveolar volatile tensions than they had when they became unconscious.

50 A **True**
    B **False**   This is part of the stress response, which is reduced by regional anaesthesia.
    C **False**   A more extensive block is needed. The block should be above T6 and may need to extend down to the lowest sacral roots for lower rectal or anal work.
    D **True**   Abolition of sympathetic supply leaves unopposed vagal innervation, reducing bowel diameter.
    E **False**   Etomidate blocks cortisol synthesis even after a single dose.

51 A **True**   To allow the stomach to be emptied.
    B **False**   Hospital stay is reduced.
    C **False**   Carbon dioxide is used. Its effect on capnography is slight.
    D **True**   Carbon dioxide is readily absorbed in the peritoneum and is mainly eliminated in the breath.
    E **False**   A head-up tilt is required to cause the abdominal contents to fall away from the gallbladder bed.

52 A **False** $(MAP - RAP) = CI \times SVRI/80$ and therefore $(MPAP - LAP) = CI \times PVRI/80$. So, $(18.5 - 10) = CI \times 241/80$. $CI = 2.82$ $l.min^{-1}.m^{-2}$.
    B **True** $(48 - 2.7) = 2.82 \times SVRI/80$. Thus $SVRI = 1285$. This is pathologically low.
    C **True**   His PCWP of 10 does not indicate adequate filling since he has some degree of ventricular depression. His cardiac output is maintained only because of his vasodilatation.
    D **True**   He probably has systemic inflammatory response syndrome (SIRS). This is most often caused by infection.
    E **False**   The ventricle is depressed, PCWP is not high and SVRI is low.

53   Regarding high-frequency jet ventilation:

A It produces low peak airway pressures.
B It seldom provides adequate carbon dioxide elimination.
C Tidal volumes should be 1–5 ml.kg^{-1}.
D It does not provide protection against aspiration of gastric contents.
E It is not useful in the spontaneously breathing patient.

54   Noradrenaline (norepinephrine):

A Inhibits the conversion of tyrosine into dihydroxyphenylalanine.
B Is broken down mainly by catechol O-methyltransferase in the presynaptic terminal.
C Is a more potent agonist at α_1 receptors than adrenaline (epinephrine).
D Causes contraction of longitudinal and circular gastrointestinal sphincters.
E Has no effect on pupil size.

55   Concerning femoral fracture:

A Analgesia is effectively provided by sciatic nerve blockade.
B Closed fracture results in 500–2000 ml of blood loss.
C It may require operation as a CEPOD class 1 emergency.
D It should be immobilised during the primary survey.
E Intramedullary nailing produces no haemodynamic compromise.

56   Regarding pulmonary oxygen toxicity:

A Pathological changes resemble those of ARDS.
B It may result in pulmonary fibrosis.
C It is a common finding in ITU patients.
D It results in death of type I pneumocytes.
E It causes alveolar oedema.

53 A **True**   This is one of its major advantages.
    B **False**   This phenomenon is not well explained by
                  conventional physiology, although it is partly
                  attributed to augmented diffusion. There may be
                  laminar flow, where exhalation occurs in an upward
                  moving layer adjacent to the tracheal wall.
    C **True**
    D **False**   There is a small but constant positive pressure in the
                  trachea – thereby providing some protection against
                  aspiration. Some clinicians do prefer to inflate the
                  cuff of an endotracheal tube in addition.
    E **False**   It is well tolerated and may facilitate weaning,
                  although it appears to suppress respiratory drive
                  somewhat.

54 A **True**   This is a negative feedback loop controlling its own
                  production.
    B **False**   Monoamine oxidase is important in the presynaptic
                  terminal.
    C **False**   Adrenaline (epinephrine) is more potent at all
                  adrenoceptors.
    D **True**   Opposing the effects of parasympathetic
                  stimulation.
    E **False**   It causes contraction of the dilator of the pupil.

55 A **False**   Femoral nerve blockade is helpful.
    B **True**   This may be virtually invisible, and bilateral fractures
                  may cause lethal haemorrhage.
    C **True**   Disruption of or pressure on the femoral artery with
                  subsequent risk to the limb may require CEPOD
                  grade 1 management.
    D **True**   This greatly reduces pain and blood loss.
    E **False**   This procedure may make the patient bleed and can
                  cause embolisation from the medulla.

56 A **True**   They resemble the changes histologically. ARDS is
                  seen in severe forms more frequently.
    B **True**   This is the end result of severe pulmonary toxicity.
    C **False**   It very rarely clinically apparent.
    D **True**   With consequent loss of surfactant. Type II cells
                  proliferate.
    E **False**   This is not seen.

57   Concerning anaesthesia for operative correction of intracranial aneurysm:

A It may require cerebral protection with deep anaesthesia.
B The anaesthetist should lower the ICP as much as possible prior to craniotomy.
C Hypotensive anaesthesia is usually required.
D It is usually performed in an asymptomatic patient.
E Venous air emboli are relatively common.

58   The following physiological changes are observed during anaesthesia:

A FRC rises slightly.
B Intra-abdominal pressure falls.
C Pulmonary shunt falls.
D Left ventricular stroke work index rises.
E Red blood cells become more rigid.

59   Causes of arterial hypoxaemia include:

A Anaemia.
B Hypoventilation.
C Low cardiac output.
D Compensated pulmonary deadspace.
E Moderate exercise.

57   A **True**   This may involve rendering the EEG isoelectric using thiopentone or etomidate.
     B **False**   This increases the aneurysmal transmural pressure gradient, potentially making it more liable to rupture.
     C **False**   It is best to maintain arterial pressure at about the same values as were recorded prior to induction.
     D **False**   It is most often performed several days after a subarachnoid haemorrhage.
     E **True**   They are much more common than in most other forms of surgery because of posture, fixed open veins and length of the procedure.

58   A **False**   It decreases, probably because of pulmonary vasodilatation and reduction in diaphragmatic and intercostal muscle tone.
     B **True**   Abdominal and diaphragmatic tone reduces.
     C **False**   It is increased, as is pulmonary deadspace fraction.
     D **False**   The cardiac ventricles are depressed, and their oxygen and glucose consumption decreases.
     E **True**   Presumably because of dissolution of volatile agent into the red cell membrane.

59   A **True**   Anaemia in the presence of a fixed pulmonary shunt causes worsening arterial hypoxaemia through desaturation of mixed venous blood.
     B **True**   Alveolar oxygen tension is reduced by hypoventilation.
     C **True**   Mixed venous desaturation in the presence of fixed shunt worsens arterial oxygenation.
     D **False**   Pulmonary deadspace may elevate alveolar carbon dioxide, reducing alveolar oxygen, but compensation will negate this effect through an increase in minute volume.
     E **False**   Arterial PO_2 typically increases during moderate exercise owing to hyperventilation.

60   Osmotic pressure:

A Is greater in a solution with large molecules.
B Is approximately 300 mosm.l^{-1} for 0.9% saline.
C Of blood is approximately 7 atm.
D Of serum is less than oncotic pressure of serum.
E Is measured by depression of freezing point.

61   Immediate preoperative preparation of the acute asthmatic patient includes:

A Bronchial dilatation.
B Corticosteroids.
C High fluid intake.
D Chromolin sodium.
E Breathing exercises.

62   Factors that can alter stimulation thresholds of pacemakers include:

A Hyperkalaemia.
B Hypokalaemia.
C Hypoxaemia.
D Catecholamines.
E Intravenous infusion of lignocaine.

63   The advantages of regional anaesthesia include:

A Decreased surgical blood loss.
B Fewer haemodynamic changes in hypertensive patients.
C Reduced incidence of thromboembolism.
D Better postoperative pain control.
E Use in patients with malignant hyperpyrexia.

60   A **False**   Osmotic pressure is determined by the
                    concentration of osmotically active particles. Their
                    size is irrelevant.
     B **False**   The osmolality is 300 mosm.l^{-1} (150 mosm.l^{-1} for
                    sodium, 150 mosm.l^{-1} for chloride). Osmotic
                    pressure is measured in units of pressure such as
                    kPa or atmospheres.
     C **True**   One mole of gas occupying one litre at standard
                    temperature has a pressure of 22.4 atmospheres
                    (Avagadro's hypothesis). Plasma osmolality =
                    300 mosm.l^{-1}, thus osmotic pressure ≈ 7 atm.
     D **False**   Osmotic pressure incorporates oncotic pressure and
                    is thus always larger. Oncotic pressure is important
                    because it is exerted by particles that cannot easily
                    leave the intravascular compartment.
     E **True**   The extent of depression is related to the amount of
                    solute.

61   A **True**
     B **False**
     C **False**
     D **False**
     E **False**
In the immediate preoperative period, only bronchial dilators
can be of some value. Corticosteroids remain controversial and
have longer onset time. Chromolin sodium is not a suitable
treatment for an acute asthma attack and therefore would be of
no value preoperatively.

62   A **True**
     B **True**
     C **True**
     D **True**
     E **True**
Other factors include myocardial ischaemia and infarction.

63   A **True**   This is due to moderate hypotension accompanying
                    regional anaesthesia.
     B **True**   Provided that intravascular volume is adequate.
     C **True**   Especially after hip replacement.
     D **True**   Particularly when regional analgesia is extended into
                    the postoperative period.
     E **True**   Avoiding known triggers of MH.

64   In the treatment of dural puncture headache:

A The use of non-steroidal anti-inflammatory drugs has revolutionised the management.
B Bedrest is nowadays not essential.
C Caffeine therapy may improve symptoms.
D Epidural blood patch has a success rate of over 90%.
E Continuous infusion of epidural saline is as good as a blood patch.

65   Calcium channel blockers have limited indications during and after CPR, which include:

A Refractory asystole.
B Electromechanical dissociation.
C Refractory ventricular tachycardia.
D Wolff–Parkinson–White syndrome.
E Hypercalcaemia.

66   A male patient of 60 years of age and known to have non insulin-dependent diabetes mellitus underwent haemorrhoidectomy in a day-case unit under general anaesthesia. In the recovery unit, his blood pressure measures about 90/60 mmHg consistently over 20 min. He is fully conscious and comfortable. Immediate management of this patient includes:

A Admission to intensive care unit for overnight observation.
B Fluid challenge with intravenous colloid and review.
C Assessment of blood loss, circulating volume and ECG.
D Insertion of internal jugular line and an arterial line.
E Inotrope infusion.

67   Pre-emptive analgesia is able to achieve the following:

A Reduced chance of developing allodynia.
B Reduced chance of developing hyperalgesia.
C Reduced requirement for analgesia in the perioperative period.
D Less chance of side effects of analgesics.
E Improvement in the quality of pain relief.

64   A **False**
      B **False**
      C **True**
      D **True**
      E **False**
Bedrest and hydration are the mainstay of initial management. The use of NSAIDs can give temporary relief but has not changed the management in a significant manner. Caffeine is a vasoconstrictor and reverses the reflex vasodilatation during spinal headache. Continuous infusion of epidural saline also produces relief, but its discontinuation causes a relapse and therefore it is not as good as an epidural blood patch.

65   A **False**
      B **False**
      C **True**
      D **False**   They can cause ventricular fibrillation in these patients.
      E **True**

66   A **False**
      B **True**
      C **True**
      D **False**
      E **False**
Immediate steps would include B and C. Steps A, D or E may be indicated on information from steps B or C, or further deterioration.

67   A **True**
      B **True**
      C **True**
      D **True**
      E **True**

68   The following can increase the incidence of residual muscle paralysis in the recovery room:

A Use of long-acting neuromuscular blockers.
B Pre-existing hypokalaemia.
C Concurrent use of narcotic agents.
D Use of thiopentone rather than propofol as induction agent.
E Hypothermia.

69   Common causes for massive postoperative haemorrhage include:

A Surgical bleeding (inadequate haemostasis).
B Primary fibrinolysis.
C Thrombocytopenia.
D Coagulation factor deficiency.
E NSAIDs.

70   The following can reflect the size of venous air embolism:

A Precordial Doppler signal.
B Decrease in end-tidal carbon dioxide.
C Increase in pulmonary arterial pressure.
D Increase in right atrial pressure.
E Mill-wheel murmur.

71   After spinal cord transection:

A Compensatory sympathetic responses below the level of injury are absent in the acute phase.
B Hyperkalaemia following suxamethonium is not seen in the first week after injury.
C The risk of hyperkalaemia following suxamethonium persists for 6 months after injury.
D Skeletal muscles tend to store twice as much potassium as normal.
E Precurarisation reliably attenuates suxamethonium-induced hyperkalaemia.

72   Regarding the effect of anaesthetic drugs:

A Minimum alveolar concentration (MAC) for volatile anaesthetics remains more or less the same in infants of all ages.
B Neonates are sensitive to opiates due to an immature blood–brain barrier.
C Infants are more sensitive to the effects of non-depolarisers than adults.
D Neonates are resistant to both depolarisers and non-depolarisers.
E The half-life of thiopentone is increased in infants when compared with older children.

68   A **True**
      B **True**
      C **False**   Narcotics have no clinically important interactions
                      with the neuromuscular blockers.
      D **False**   While the choice of induction agent can influence
                      the onset of action it has no significant effect on the
                      duration of action of muscle relaxants.
      E **True**

69   A **True**
      B **False**
      C **False**
      D **False**
      E **False**
      B, C and D will manifest intraoperatively and are unlikely to be
      the cause of massive haemorrhage. NSAIDs are more likely to
      cause generalised oozing rather than massive haemorrhage.

70   A **False**   This device indicates the presence of air bubbles but
                      it cannot measure the size.
      B **True**
      C **True**
      D **True**
      E **True**

71   A **True**
      B **False**   It can be seen within 72 h of injury.
      C **True**
      D **False**   The reason for suxamethonium-induced
                      hyperkalaemia is proliferation of cholinergic
                      receptors on the muscle surface.
      E **False**   None of the methods is reliable.

72   A **False**   MAC at birth is 25% less than the adult value. It
                      gradually increases up to 3 months.
      B **True**
      C **True**
      D **False**   The neuromuscular junction is not fully developed
                      up to 3 months of age. This causes resistance to
                      depolarisers and sensitivity to non-depolarisers.
      E **True**   This is because of diminished hepatic and renal
                      clearance.

73   Characteristic features of fetal circulation are:

A High systemic vascular resistance.
B Low pulmonary vascular resistance.
C Right to left shunt through ductus arteriosus.
D Right to left shunt through foramen ovale.
E Umbilical artery has less oxygenated blood than umbilical vein.

74   In valvular heart disease:

A Aortic valve area of less than 2 cm² is abnormal.
B Pulse pressure is increased with aortic stenosis.
C Decrease in heart rate increases regurgitation in aortic incompetence.
D Mitral valve area of less than 2 cm² produces significant symptoms.
E Surgery is not indicated unless the patient is symptomatic at rest.

75   Factors that predispose to digitalis toxicity are:

A Hypokalaemia.
B Hypercalcaemia.
C Hypermagnesaemia.
D Hyperventilation.
E Renal failure.

76   In a patient with essential hypertension:

A Decrease in blood pressure during anaesthesia is more likely than in a normotensive patient.
B Adequate control of preoperative blood pressure ensures a lack of intraoperative hypertension.
C There is a lack of cerebral blood flow autoregulation.
D Preoperative diastolic blood pressure must be less than 90 mmHg.
E A routine preoperative ECG is not appropriate.

77   Possible causes of hypotension following carotid artery surgery include:

A Denervation of carotid sinus.
B Plaque removal from the region of the baroreceptor.
C Transection of recurrent laryngeal nerve.
D Trauma to the stellate ganglion.
E Hypovolaemia.

73 A **False**   The placenta has a low-resistance vascular system.
    B **False**   As the lungs are not inflated, the vascular resistance is high.
    C **True**
    D **True**
    E **True**   The umbilical vein carries oxygenated blood from the placenta.

74 A **True**   Normal values range from 2.6 to 3.5 cm². Surgery should be performed if the area is reduced to 0.8 cm².
    B **False**   It is reduced in aortic stenosis and is increased in aortic regurgitation.
    C **True**   Decreased heart rate results in increased diastolic time and, therefore, regurgitation.
    D **True**   Normal area is 4–6 cm². Less than 1.1 cm² is critical and produces pulmonary oedema.
    E **False**   Surgery should ideally be performed before this stage.

75 A **True**
    B **True**
    C **False**   Hypomagnesaemia is known to predispose to digitalis toxicity.
    D **True**   Hyperventilation causes hypokalaemia.
    E **True**   Digitalis is excreted principally by the kidneys.

76 A **True**   Hypertensive patients, despite adequate control of blood pressure, are more prone to both hypertensive and hypotensive episodes in the perioperative period.
    B **False**   The incidence is reduced but intraoperative hypertension can still occur.
    C **False**   The autoregulation occurs at a higher range of blood pressure.
    D **False**   Desirable but not a must.
    E **False**   All hypertensive patients should have a preoperative ECG.

77 A **False**   This would cause hypertension.
    B **True**   Plaque removal increases baroreceptor sensitivity.
    C **False**
    D **False**
    E **True**

78   Following a needlestick injury from a patient with hepatitis:

A 30% of hepatitis B exposed individuals are likely to become infected.
B 90% of hepatitis C exposed individuals are likely to be infected.
C Vaccination should be received within 48 h of exposure to a patient with hepatitis A.
D Vaccination should be received within 1 month of exposure to a patient with hepatitis C.
E High anti-hepatitis B surface antigen titre immune globulin (HBIG) is recommended in healthcare workers who have no antibodies to hepatitis B surface antigen.

79   In the management of the brain-stem dead organ donor:

A Intravascular volume and cardiac output should be optimised.
B α agonists are ideal to maintain blood pressure.
C Dopamine and dobutamine are of little value.
D Diuretics or mannitol should not be used to correct oliguria.
E Warm-ischaemia time should be kept to a minimum.

80   Among diuretics:

A Carbonic anhydrase inhibitors act on the proximal tubule.
B Carbonic anhydrase inhibitors cause hypochloraemia and hypokalaemia.
C Spironolactone inhibits the action of aldosterone.
D Thiazides act on the proximal tubule.
E Mannitol inhibits chloride reabsorption in the ascending limb.

78 A **True**
    B **False**   Hepatitis C has a low profile of infectivity. 3–5% of
                   exposed individuals eventually become infected.
    C **False**   No vaccine is available. Immune globulins provide
                   passive immunity.
    D **False**   No vaccine is available.
    E **True**

79 A **True**
    B **False**   These may reduce organ blood flow.
    C **False**   These are often required to optimise organ blood
                   flow.
    D **False**   These may need to be administered to facilitate
                   urine output.
    E **True**

80 A **True**
    B **False**   Hyperchloraemia.
    C **True**
    D **False**   They act on the distal convoluted tubule.
    E **False**   This is the action of loop diuretics.

Paper 3

81 **Regarding patients' preoperative use of recreational drugs:**

A Opioid abuse often results in euphoria, constipation and opioid sensitivity.
B Cocaine abuse may cause postoperative convulsions.
C Drug abuse always causes increased resistance to anaesthetic drugs.
D Cannabis abuse results in no discernible chronic symptoms.
E Amphetamine abuse causes neurosis but not psychosis.

82 **Regarding preoperative scoring systems:**

A American Society of Anesthesiologists (ASA) grading correlates with perioperative risk of death.
B A patient with ASA grade 4 has a disease that is not incapacitating.
C ASA grading, although specific, is insensitive.
D APACHE III scoring may be useful in perioperative risk management.
E Paucity of adverse perioperative events aids design of such scoring systems.

83 **Regarding chronic liver disease:**

A It often causes hypoxaemia.
B It results in an elevated cardiac output and reduced systemic vascular resistance.
C Severe secondary pulmonary hypertension may develop.
D Hepatic flow–metabolism coupling is better under isoflurane anaesthesia than under regional anaesthesia.
E Hyperkalaemia is common.

84 **Regarding anti-arrhythmic drugs:**

A Calcium channel blockers prolong atrioventricular node refractoriness.
B Verapamil should not be used in Wolff–Parkinson–White syndrome.
C Phenytoin is useful in treating digitalis toxicity because it enhances nodal conduction.
D Amiodarone is a β-blocker.
E Bretylium magnifies the effects of exogenous catecholamines but reduces the effects of indirect sympathomimetics.

Answers

81 A **False**   These patients are usually resistant to opioids.
    B **True**
    C **False**   Some drugs of abuse reduce anaesthetic requirements.
    D **False**   Memory loss, anxiety, panic attacks and low motivation are among the more common symptoms.
    E **False**   Amphetamines and cocaine may cause psychosis.

82 A **True**   Although the correlation is weak and it allows no identification of factors.
    B **False**   ASA 4 grading indicates a disease that is a constant threat to life.
    C **False**   ASA grading is non-specific.
    D **True**   Few trials have been conducted, however.
    E **False**   Paucity of adverse events makes design difficult.

83 A **True**   Intrapulmonary shunting increases and hypoxic pulmonary vasoconstriction is impaired.
    B **True**
    C **True**   This may be a contraindication to liver transplant.
    D **False**   Although isoflurane preserves it better than halothane or enflurane.
    E **False**   Hypokalaemia is common due to hyperaldosteronism.

84 A **True**
    B **True**   It may shorten the refractoriness of the accessory pathway and increase the ventricular response rate.
    C **True**
    D **True**   It is also an α-blocker.
    E **True**   This is because it depletes terminals and blocks reuptake.

85   Concerning premedication in children:

A Phenothiazines are a popular premedicant.

B Benzodiazepines produce dangerously unpredictable sedation in children, and should not be used.

C Oral anticholinergic premedication is ineffective because of its poor intestinal absorption.

D Thiopentone 40 mg.kg^{-1} given rectally produces satisfactory preoperative conditions.

E Sedative premedication is helpful in the anxious patient presenting for emergency surgery.

86   Regarding pulse oximetry:

A Pulse oximetry is sensitive to changes in high values of arterial oxygen tension.

B The pulse oximeter uses two monochromatic light-emitting diodes.

C The isobestic point of haemoglobin and deoxyhaemoglobin is the ideal wavelength for pulse oximetry.

D Weighted averaging improves accuracy but introduces lag into measurement.

E Ambient light is measured many times per second.

87   Regarding the monitoring of coagulation:

A Bleeding time measures the effectiveness of platelets and is usually $3\frac{1}{2}$–$8\frac{1}{2}$ min.

B The thrombin time tests the common pathway.

C Measurement of activated clotting time (ACT) requires an activator and is usually 105–167 s.

D Thromboelastography examines the entire process of clot formation rather than static, isolated functions.

E Activated partial thromboplastin time (APTT) assesses the intrinsic pathway and is raised during cardiopulmonary bypass.

88   Benzodiazepines:

A May produce phlebitis.

B Produce anaphylactic reactions less frequently than barbiturates.

C May be reversed using flumazenil, although its β half-life is shorter than that of any benzodiazepine.

D Do not cause loss of the eyelash reflex on induction of anaesthesia.

E Produce greater amnesia than propofol when used for induction of anaesthesia.

85 A **True**
    B **False**
    C **False**   Quaternary amines, such as glycopyrrolate, are poorly absorbed but tertiary amines, such as atropine, are adequately absorbed and may be given orally.
    D **True**   This regime is not often used since more intense observation is required after administration.
    E **False**   Most patients presenting as emergencies should not be sedated preoperatively.

86 A **False**   It is particularly insensitive.
    B **True**   One at 660 nm and one at 940 nm.
    C **False**   It is the point at which both absorb the same amount of light, and is 805 nm. It is thus not useful.
    D **True**
    E **True**   In the UK, 400 times per second.

87 A **True**
    B **True**
    C **True**   The usual activator is diatomaceous earth but this is affected by aprotonin.
    D **True**
    E **True**

88 A **True**   Diazepam (before being prepared as an emulsion – Diazemuls™) frequently caused phlebitis.
    B **True**
    C **True**   If effective, it should be followed by an infusion to prevent re-sedation.
    D **False**   They do, in common with the barbiturates.
    E **True**   The duration of amnesia produced is much longer.

89   Regarding the maintenance of anaesthesia:

A The 'minimum infusion rate' (MIR) is the infusion rate of an i.v. anaesthetic that prevents movement in response to skin incision in 50% of patients.

B The ED_{95} of propofol (as the sole anaesthetic) is approximately 350 μg.kg.min^{-1}.

C The ED_{95} to ED_{50} ratio for propofol is more than 2.

D The ED_{50} for isoflurane is 1.16%. The ED_{95} is 1.63%.

E At 1 minimum alveolar concentration (MAC) equivalent 50% of patients are unaware of a standard skin incision.

90   Regarding intestinal anastomoses:

A Postoperative leak is significantly greater when morphine is used for analgesia than when pethidine is used.

B Anastomotic leak is caused by reduced bowel blood flow.

C Epidural opioids affect intestinal activity.

D Halothane abolishes all intestinal activity.

E Choice of anaesthetic and analgesic technique is the single most important factor in determining whether an anastomosis will leak.

91   Regarding patients with phaeochromocytoma:

A Clonidine is an effective agent for preoperative preparation.

B Atropine premedication is recommended.

C 10% of tumours are benign.

D Diagnosis may be suspected on finding elevated levels of 5-hydroxyindoleacetic acid in the urine.

E Postoperative hyperglycaemia is caused by the abrupt withdrawal of elevated catecholamine levels.

92   The following data are obtained from a patient with a pulmonary artery catheter in situ: inspired oxygen fraction 0.21, cardiac index 3 l.min^{-1}.m^{-2}, arterial oxygen saturation 85%, arterial oxygen tension 9.54 kPa, mixed venous oxygen saturation 48.5%, mixed venous oxygen tension 5.24 kPa, haemoglobin 145 g.l^{-1}.

A The arterial oxyhaemoglobin saturation curve is shifted to the left.

B Acidosis may explain the shift of the oxyhaemoglobin saturation curve.

C Oxygen delivery index is 401 ml.min^{-1}m^{-2}.

D The patient has a normal metabolic rate.

E A fall in cardiac output may cause the arterial oxygen tension to rise.

89 A **True**   It corresponds to MAC.
    B **True**
    C **True**   This has serious implications for the risk of
                     awareness with i.v. anaesthesia.
    D **True**   Note that the ED_{95} to ED_{50} ratio is much smaller than
                     for propofol.
    E **False**   The definition of MAC uses movement response.

90 A **False**
    B **True**   This causes tissue death and anastomotic
                     breakdown.
    C **True**   They have been implicated in increasing
                     anastomotic breakdown rates.
    D **True**   This inhibition persists even in the presence of
                     neostigmine.
    E **False**   Surgical technique, the patient's general condition
                     and the presence of infection are much more
                     important.

91 A **False**   This is an α_2 agonist, and is ineffective in
                     preoperative preparation.
    B **False**   This can cause serious tachyarrhythmias.
    C **False**   10% of tumours are malignant.
    D **False**   Carcinoid syndrome is detected in this manner.
    E **False**   Hypoglycaemia may ensue.

92 A **False**   It is shifted to the right. An oxygen tension of
                     9.54 kPa would normally result in a saturation of
                     approximately 94%.
    B **True**   A respiratory or metabolic acidosis could cause this.
    C **False** $DO_2I = CI \times (SaO_2 \times Hb \times 1.34 + PaO_2 \times 0.2)$. $DO_2I = 3 \times$
                     $(165.2 + 1.9)$. $DO_2I = 501$ ml.min^{-1}.m^{-2}.
    D **False** VO_2I = arterial DO_2I – venous DO_2I. $VO_2I = 501 - 286 =$
                     215 ml.min^{-1}.m^{-2}. This is elevated from the normal
                     rate of 136 ml.min^{-1}.m^{-2}.
    E **False**   A fall in cardiac output will further desaturate the
                     mixed venous blood, causing shunting of more
                     desaturated blood, causing further hypoxaemia.

93   Weaning from mechanical ventilation:

A May improve cor pulmonale.
B Is unlikely if forced vital capacity is less than 10 ml.kg^{-1}.
C Is faster using pressure-assisted/supported spontaneous ventilation than using any other method.
D Is occasionally delayed by hyperphosphataemia.
E Is not dependent upon the resting respiratory minute volume.

94   Concerning Student's *t*-test:

A It was described by a student.
B It is useful in analysing non-parametric data.
C It should be used as a one-tailed test wherever possible.
D A paired test may be used if the two sample groups are of equal sizes.
E It requires that the population conforms to a normal distribution.

95   A 26-year-old man has sustained severe blunt injury to the anterior thorax.

A Muffled heart sounds should prompt immediate pericardiocentesis.
B Hypoxaemia is most likely to be due to hypoventilation.
C ECG monitoring is mandatory.
D Pulmonary contusion is likely to be present.
E Thoracic aortic disruption may typically be recognised as anterior chest pain.

96   Systemic inflammatory response syndrome:

A Usually presents as maldistributive shock with a low systemic vascular resistance.
B Always demonstrates a hyperdynamic circulation.
C Is due to systemic release of prostaglandins.
D Has a 90% mortality.
E Should be treated with corticosteroids.

93 A **True**   The reduction in pulmonary vascular resistance removes some of the impediment to right ventricular ejection.

B **True**   The FVC should be above 15 ml.kg^{-1} before weaning is commenced.

C **False**   No single method has been shown to be consistently superior.

D **False**   Hypophosphataemia is occasionally implicated in producing a delay through respiratory muscle weakness.

E **False**   A resting minute volume of 10 l.min^{-1} or more is associated with failure to wean.

94 A **False**   It was described by W.S. Gossett, a Dublin brewery worker. He submitted it under the name 'Student' because employees were not allowed to publish the results of their work.

B **False**   It is used to analyse normally distributed data.

C **False**   A one-tailed test examines differences in one direction only and is rarely called for.

D **False**   A paired test may only be used when the data themselves are paired.

E **True**   See B.

95 A **False**   Clinical signs of a dangerous tamponade should prompt immediate pericardiocentesis, but a finding of just muffled heart sounds does not prompt such a dangerous procedure.

B **False**   It is most likely to be due to pulmonary contusion, haemorrhage or low cardiac output.

C **True**   Arrhythmias are common.

D **True**   Even quite minor thoracic injuries produce some pulmonary contusion, causing hypoxaemia through shunting.

E **False**   It more typically presents as pain in the upper back. Lack of pain here does not exclude it, however.

96 A **False**   It usually presents as hypovolaemic shock, which upon correction becomes maldistributive.

B **False**   See A.

C **False**   It is due to a pantheon of endogenous chemicals, but prostaglandins do not play a major role.

D **False**   Mortality is significantly better, and is dependent upon other pathology, stage, severity and aetiology.

E **False**   This may worsen the prognosis if the cause is infective.

97   Regarding the laryngeal mask:

A It provides no protection of the airway from soiling by gastric contents.
B It may be used for tonsillectomy.
C A size 5 laryngeal mask is suitable for small children.
D It has a role in resuscitation.
E It should be disposed of after one use.

98   Concerning temperature regulation during anaesthesia:

A Hypothalamic control of temperature is impaired.
B The majority of heat loss occurs via the breathing system.
C Most patients leave the operating theatre with a core temperature below 36°C.
D Hypothermia causes a fall in urine output.
E Metabolic rate falls by 10% for each 1°C fall in temperature.

99   During mechanical ventilation of the lungs, doubling the respiratory rate while keeping the tidal volume constant will:

A Increase anatomical deadspace.
B Halve the $PvCO_2$.
C Reduce venous return to the heart.
D Increase mean inspiratory pressure.
E Reduce FRC.

100   Left ventricular stroke work index:

A Is increased by adrenaline.
B Is measured in joules.
C Is affected only by contractility and preload.
D Is defined as: stroke volume × afterload.
E May be measured using a pulmonary artery catheter.

101   The following can assist in the management of postoperative stridor:

A Assisted respiration.
B Humidified oxygen therapy.
C Racemic adrenaline.
D Bronchodilators.
E Antibiotics.

97 A **True**
    B **True**   It has been used successfully.
    C **False**   Size 5 is the largest currently available. Sizes 1–3 are
                    suitable for children.
    D **True**   It is easy to place in an adequate position and thus
                    may be useful when personnel trained in tracheal
                    intubation are not available.
    E **False**   Laryngeal masks are multi-use devices and are
                    sterilised between uses. If used many times, they
                    eventually perish and must be replaced.

98 A **True**   A new, lower set point is made.
    B **False**   Only a very small amount is lost this way. Most is
                    lost through convection from exposed areas,
                    especially via the open abdomen or thorax.
    C **True**
    D **False**   The urine flow rate is maintained because the ability
                    of the kidney to conserve water is impaired.
    E **False**   It falls by approximately 6–8% per °C.

99 A **False**   This will have no effect.
    B **False**   The $PaCO_2$ will be approximately halved, but the
                    addition of carbon dioxide to the capillary blood is
                    unchanged, so $PvCO_2$ will be reduced but will be
                    greater than half of its original value, assuming
                    unchanged cardiac output.
    C **True**   There will be a net increase in pulmonary vascular
                    resistance, reducing left ventricular venous return.
    D **True**   Increasing the respiratory rate will prevent complete
                    exhalation, increasing the mean intrathoracic
                    volume, increasing mean inspiratory pressure.
    E **False**   FRC may increase, see D.

100 A **True**   The afterload and the contractility increase.
    B **False**   It is measured in $g.m.m^{-2}$.
    C **False**   It is affected by contractility, preload and afterload.
    D **False**   LVSWI = (MAP − PCWP) × SV × 0.0136.
    E **True**   This is the most common way of measuring it.

101 A **True**   Especially if the stridor is inspiratory.
    B **True**   This will improve oxygenation.
    C **True**   This reduces the mucosal congestion.
    D **True**   Improving oxygenation and reducing respiratory
                    work.
    E **False**
    Steroids are controversial. Patients should be closely followed
    after receiving racemic adrenaline as rebound can occur.

102 Severe vomiting from pyloric stenosis in a 2-month-old child could result in:

A Arterial pH of 7.16.
B Daily urine output of 400 ml.
C High, peakedT waves on electrocardiogram.
D Serum chloride level of 78 ml/l.
E Dehydration.

103 Local anaesthetic deposited in the epidural space can produce its effect by the following means:

A Action on the dorsal ganglion.
B Action after systemic absorption.
C Action on spinal roots as they exit from the cord.
D Action on dural cuffs.
E Action on spinal nerves in paravertebral spaces.

104 Ethyl alcohol affects its blocking action by:

A Interfering with the release of neurotransmitters.
B Suppressing mitochondrial activity.
C Calcium channel block.
D Sodium channel block.
E Denervation of nerve fibres and precipitation of proteins.

105 Regarding adrenergic agonists:

A Dobutamine is the next inotrope choice after adrenaline to support the beating heart in the CPR setting.
B Catecholamine cardiomyopathy is a risk with isoprenaline treatment.
C Dopamine requires correction of severe metabolic acidosis for its optimal effect.
D Isoprenaline shunts blood away from vital organs.
E Noradrenaline can be the last resort in pharmacological support of the ischaemic heart.

102 A **False**
     B **False**   Urine output is reduced due to dehydration.
     C **False**   High, peaked T waves are characteristic of
                     hyperkalaemia.
     D **True**
     E **True**
Persistent vomiting results in the loss of hydrogen ions from the
stomach. As hydrogen ions are lost, the kidneys secrete
potassium in exchange for hydrogen ions in an effort to maintain
a normal arterial pH. In addition, the kidneys begin exchanging
potassium and hydrogen ions for sodium ions as the infant
becomes sodium depleted from vomiting. The result is a
dehydrated infant with a hypokalaemic, hypochloraemic,
metabolic alkalosis.

103 A **True**
     B **False**   This reduces the availability of local anaesthetic.
     C **True**
     D **True**
     E **True**
Local anaesthetic deposited in the epidural space can spread
anywhere from spinal cord to dorsal ganglion. Its systemic
absorption can produce systemic but not regional effects.

104 A **False**
     B **False**
     C **False**
     D **False**
     E **True**
Ethyl alcohol acts on the plasma membrane and destroys its
structure by precipitating the proteins. This leads to denervation.

105 A **False**   The answer is dopamine. Dobutamine can cause
                     vasodilatation and hypotension and thus can worsen
                     the outcome in the CPR setting.
     B **True**   Isoprenaline also causes a rapid downregulation of
                     β receptors.
     C **True**   So does noradrenaline.
     D **True**   This is due to profound vasodilatation in muscular
                     beds.
     E **True**   It may increase diastolic blood pressure and thus
                     coronary blood flow.

106 Common postoperative problems that lead to unexpected hospital admission following day-case surgery are:

A Pain.
B Persistent nausea and vomiting.
C Fluctuating blood pressure.
D Failure to regain consciousness.
E Unresolving conduction block.

107 Incidence of respiratory depression after spinal opioids is increased by the following factors:

A Old age.
B Concurrent use of benzodiazepines.
C Coughing and straining.
D Use of lipophilic opioids.
E Subarachnoid rather than epidural route of administration.

108 Possible causes of stridor in the recovery room after thyroidectomy include:

A Residual paralysis.
B Surgical bleeding.
C Bilateral recurrent laryngeal nerve paralysis.
D Hypercalcaemia.
E Wound infection causing swelling of the neck.

109 Cerebral blood flow (CBF) is increased by:

A Increased level of carbon dioxide in the blood.
B 1 MAC of halothane.
C Moderate hypothermia.
D Etomidate.
E Ketamine.

110 Complications of venous air embolism include:

A Acute cor pulmonale.
B Pulmonary oedema.
C Myocardial ischaemia secondary to paradoxical emboli in coronary vasculature.
D Refractory hypoxaemia.
E Bronchospasm.

106 A **True**
     B **True**
     C **True**
     D **False**   Theoretically possible but not a common
                     postoperative problem in day-case units.
     E **True**

107 A **True**
     B **True**
     C **True**   Causing cephalad spread of drugs in the CSF.
     D **False**   Hydrophilic opioids are more likely to stay unbound
                     and, therefore, are more likely to spread.
     E **True**

108 A **True**
     B **True**   Sutures should be cut immediately to release the
                     pressure in the wound.
     C **True**
     D **False**   Hypocalcaemia is more likely if the parathyroids
                     have also been removed.
     E **False**   It is too early for infection to manifest.

109 A **True**
     B **True**   Volatile anaesthetics administered during
                     normocapnia to produce an MAC > 0.6 cause
                     dose-dependent increase in CBF. Halothane
                     > enflurane > isoflurane.
     C **False**   Hypothermia reduces cerebral metabolic rate.
     D **False**   All intravenous anaesthetics (except ketamine)
                     reduce cerebral metabolism as well as CBF.
     E **True**

110 A **True**
     B **True**   This is due to an increase in pulmonary arterial
                     pressure.
     C **True**   This occurs in patients with patent foramen ovale.
     D **True**
     E **True**

111   **Typical anatomical features of a neonatal airway are:**

A Narrow nares.
B Large pharynx.
C Large tongue.
D Fixed epiglottis.
E High, anterior and tapered larynx with maximal narrowing at the true vocal cords.

112   **The following features are characteristic of acute epiglottitis:**

A Children less than 2 years of age.
B Expiratory stridor.
C Narrowing of the subglottic area in neck X-ray.
D Fever, neutrophilia and drooling.
E Rapid onset with symptoms developed over the last 24 h.

113   **Fetal haemoglobin has an increased affinity for oxygen and this results in:**

A P_{50} of 19 mmHg.
B Greater uptake of oxygen.
C Increased release of oxygen to tissues.
D Shift of the oxyhaemoglobin dissociation curve to the left.
E Physiological anaemia at 3 months of age.

114   **Ventricular wall stress:**

A Is increased with increase in wall thickness.
B Is increased with increased intraventricular pressure.
C Is increased with increased radius of the chamber.
D Reduces coronary perfusion.
E Increases oxygen consumption.

115   **Appropriate emergency management of cardiac tamponade associated with severely compromised haemodynamics will include:**

A Pericardiocentesis under general anaesthesia.
B Swan–Ganz catheter for pressure monitoring.
C Fluids and inotropes to normalise haemodynamics before undertaking pericardiocentesis.
D Echocardiography for correct assessment of the amount of pericardial fluid.
E Vasodilators to improve cardiac output by reducing the afterload.

111 A **True**
     B **False**   The pharynx is relatively small.
     C **True**
     D **False**   The epiglottis is mobile.
     E **False**   Maximal narrowing is at the cricoid cartilage, whereas in adults the maximal narrowing is usually at the true cords.

112 A **False**   Typically it is seen in children between 2 and 6 years of age. Croup is more common under 2 years of age.
     B **False**   Inspiratory stridor is characteristic.
     C **False**   This is seen in croup. In epiglottitis, the lateral view of the neck shows swelling of the epiglottis and aryepiglottic fold.
     D **True**
     E **True**

113 A **True**   The oxyhaemoglobin dissociation (OHD) curve is shifted to the left.
     B **True**   Caused by the shift of the OHD curve.
     C **False**   Oxygen release to the tissues is greater with a right-shifted OHD curve.
     D **True**
     E **True**   This is when more and more of the HbF is replaced by HbA.

114 A **False**   Wall stress (Laplace's law) = intraventricular pressure $\times$ radius $\times$ wall thickness^{-1}. Increase in the wall thickness may be compensatory to reduce the stress.
     B **True**
     C **True**
     D **True**
     E **True**

115 A **False**   Local anaesthesia is more appropriate for pericardiocentesis in a patient with severely compromised haemodynamics.
     B **False**   The priority is to perform pericardiocentesis. Pressure monitoring is unlikely to influence immediate management.
     C **False**   Fluids and inotropes are given while pericardiocentesis is awaited. It is not appropriate to try to normalise haemodynamics, as it may not be an achievable aim under the circumstances.
     D **False**   Echocardiography aids correct placement of the pericardiocentesis needle but it is of no use to make a correct assessment of the volume of fluid in these circumstances.
     E **False**   Vasodilators will produce severe hypotension.

116 Appropriate measures to prevent the hypertensive response to laryngoscopy in hypertensive patients include:

A Precurarisation.
B Administration of alfentanil or fentanyl prior to induction of anaesthesia.
C Intravenous lignocaine prior to induction of anaesthesia.
D Intravenous propranolol prior to induction of anaesthesia.
E Increasing the dose of induction agent to 1.5–2 times normal.

117 In the treatment of myocardial ischaemia associated with hypotension:

A Nitroglycerine or nifedipine will inevitably cure the problem.
B Intravenous fluids are contraindicated, as they will worsen the situation.
C Inotropes should not be given, as they will increase ischaemia.
D Vasoconstrictors have no role.
E Invasive monitoring should not be undertaken as this may cause arrhythmias.

118 With regard to liver function tests:

A Alanine aminotransferase (ALT) is more specific than aspartate aminotransferase (AST).
B Elevated alkaline phosphatase (ALP) indicates primarily hepatocellular injury.
C Prothrombin time is a sensitive indicator for acute hepatocellular injury.
D All clotting factors except factor VIII are synthesised by the liver.
E Serum albumin is reduced within 48 h of acute injury to the liver.

119 Reperfusion injury in the transplanted organ:

A Is seen during re-establishment of blood flow to a previously ischaemic organ.
B Is not seen after liver transplant.
C Is related to production of oxygen-derived free radicals.
D Is caused by oxidation of lipids, proteins and nucleic acids.
E Can be suppressed in the presence of high-energy substrates.

120 Mannitol has the following effects:

A Reduction of intracranial pressure.
B Increased renal blood flow.
C Increased tubular flow.
D Free radical scavenging.
E Improvement in symptoms of heart failure.

116 A **False**   Precurarisation reduces suxamethonium induced
                     side effects.
     B **True**   This is a central effect and is due to deeper levels of
                     anaesthesia.
     C **True**   Probably due to a central effect, and to direct
                     vasodilatation and myocardial depression.
     D **False**   A short-acting alternative such as esmolol is
                     appropriate.
     E **False**   It may be effective but is not appropriate.

117 A **False**
     B **False**
     C **False**
     D **False**
     E **False**
Monitoring of filling pressure and calculation of systemic
vascular resistance will allow logical intervention. Intravenous
fluids will help if filling pressure is low. Inotropes + nitroglycerine
may help if filling pressure is high. Excessively reduced vascular
resistance is an indication for vasoconstrictors and an increased
vascular resistance is an indication for vasodilators.

118 A **True**   AST is also secreted by the pancreas, muscles, heart
                     and red blood cells.
     B **False**   ALP is more specific for hepatobiliary disease and an
                     obstructive pattern.
     C **True**
     D **True**
     E **False**   Serum albumin takes a few days before its
                     concentration starts falling.

119 A **True**
     B **False**
     C **True**
     D **True**
     E **False**   High-energy substrates enhance the injury.

120 A **True**   Only if vascular integrity is present.
     B **True**   Due to increased cardiac output and reduced renal
                     vascular resistance.
     C **True**   Osmotic diuresis.
     D **True**
     E **False**   It increases preload and therefore worsens heart
                     failure.

Paper 4

121 Concerning cigarette smoking by patients:

A It is associated with worse postoperative outcome.

B It causes some monitors to give unreliable readings.

C Risk is reduced to that of a non-smoker if smoking is stopped for 12 h or more.

D Abstention for 6–8 weeks is required to repair the mucociliary staircase.

E Smokers' operations should be postponed, as most will stop smoking if instructed by the anaesthetist.

122 Concerning the prediction and grading of difficulty in airway management:

A Mallampati described a four-point system to predict difficulty in intubation.

B Mallampati scoring is the most sensitive predictor of difficulty in intubation.

C A thyromental distance of 5 cm or more is associated with difficulty in airway management.

D The glottis is invisible in a Cormack and Lehane grade 3.

E Mandibular recession is not, in isolation, associated with difficulty in airway management.

123 Regarding carcinoid syndrome:

A Carcinoid tumours are found in the small bowel, bronchi and ovaries.

B Bowel carcinoid tumours are less likely per se to cause carcinoid syndrome.

C Carcinoid syndrome is caused by the release of serotonin, histamine, prostaglandins and kallikreins.

D Regurgitant or stenotic valvular heart defects may result.

E Hypoglycaemia is often seen during acute episodes.

Answers

---

121 A **True**   Pulmonary and myocardial events are more common.
     B **True**   Pulse oximetry may read falsely high.
     C **False**   The risk may never be reversed since permanent damage may have occurred.
     D **True**
     E **False**   Few patients will stop smoking after instruction by the anaesthetist.

122 A **False**   Mallampati described a three-point system, to which Samsoon and Young added a fourth point.
     B **False**   Previous difficulty is the best predictor of future difficulty.
     C **False**   Short thyromental distances are associated with difficulty.
     D **True**   Only the epiglottis is visible.
     E **False**

123 A **True**
     B **True**   Substances released by bowel tumours pass through the liver before reaching the systemic circulation.
     C **True**   Kallikreins stimulate the production of bradykinin.
     D **True**   Tricuspid regurgitation and pulmonary stenosis are relatively common.
     E **False**   Hyperglycaemia is seen.

124 Concerning cardiac glycosides:

A They reduce the cardiac action potential duration.
B They increase vagal tone, increasing conduction through the atrioventricular node.
C They enhance automaticity by increasing the rate of phase 4 depolarisation.
D Digoxin toxicity may be treated by i.v. administration of potassium.
E Positive inotropic effect is mediated by inhibition of the Na^+-Ca^{2+} pump.

125 Regarding premedication:

A Opioid premedication reduces serum catecholamine levels.
B Opioid premedication reduces the risk of aspiration pneumonitis.
C Atropine premedication reduces the risk of aspiration pneumonitis.
D Opioid premedication is desirable before ophthalmic surgery.
E Subcutaneous premedication is more reliably absorbed than intramuscular premedication.

126 Regarding inaccuracy in pulse oximetry:

A Methaemoglobinaemia drives the measured saturation towards 85%.
B To differentiate between the various species of haemoglobin, light of wavelength less than 550 nm is required.
C Carboxyhaemoglobin absorbs light strongly at 660 nm but weakly at 940 nm.
D Jaundice causes inaccuracy in measuring saturation.
E Valve defects may cause spurious hypoxaemia.

127 Regarding therapeutic indices:

A The therapeutic index is the fatal dose in 50% of patients divided by the therapeutic dose in 50% of patients.
B The therapeutic index of barbiturate induction agents is approximately 4–6.
C The therapeutic index of midazolam is 12–15.
D Steroidal anaesthetic drugs have lower therapeutic indices than the barbiturates.
E Propofol has a similar therapeutic margin to the barbiturates.

124 A **True**   This is a pro-arrhythmic action.
    B **False**   They increase vagal tone, slowing AV nodal
                   conduction.
    C **True**   This is also a pro-arrhythmic action.
    D **True**   Toxicity may be treated this way in the hypokalaemic
                  patient, but digoxin occasionally produces
                  hyperkalaemia, so care must be exercised.
    E **False**   The positive inotropic effect is mediated by inhibiting
                   the Na^+–K^+ pump, increasing intracellular Na^+, thus
                   increasing Na^+–Ca^{2+} exchange at the cell surface, and
                   elevating intracellular Ca^{2+} concentration.

125 A **False**   Carbon dioxide retention often elevates serum
                   catecholamine levels.
    B **False**   The delay in gastric emptying may make aspiration
                   pneumonitis more likely.
    C **False**   There is no evidence of an effect in either direction.
                   Gastric emptying is delayed, but acid secretion is
                   reduced.
    D **False**   This may result in raised intraocular pressure
                   through vomiting.
    E **False**   Intramuscular blood supply is more predictable.

126 A **True**   This is irrespective of the actual saturation.
    B **True**   These wavelengths are absorbed by skin and so
                  such oximetry is limited to in vitro.
    C **True**
    D **False**
    E **True**   Tricuspid regurgitation may cause marked venous
                  pulsatility.

127 A **False**   This is defined in animals rather than patients.
    B **True**
    C **False**   It is 4–6.
    D **False**   They are relatively safer in overdose.
    E **True**

128 Ketamine:

A Is a racemic mixture.
B Is derived from phencyclidine.
C Blocks both uptake-1 and uptake-2 reuptake mechanisms of noradrenaline.
D Is a drug of abuse, being used recreationally.
E Produces some emergence phenomena, which may be treated by distraction and re-sedation.

129 Concerning i.v. maintenance of anaesthesia:

A It is better when calculated using lean body mass than total body mass.
B For i.v. maintenance, steady-state infusion rate = steady-state plasma concentration × clearance.
C Constant rate infusion takes 4–5 times the redistribution half-life of the drug to reach steady state.
D The 95% confidence interval of the ED_{95} of propofol is similar in size to that of isoflurane.
E Administration of 67% nitrous oxide reduces the required plasma concentration of propofol for anaesthesia by over 50%.

130 Regarding colonic blood flow:

A Isoflurane increases splanchnic vascular resistance.
B Loss of 10% of circulating blood volume causes an 80% drop in splanchnic blood flow.
C Morphine increases colonic tone and reduces splanchnic blood flow.
D Vasoconstriction in the splanchnic circulation is more sensitive to hypovolaemia than that in skeletal muscles.
E Fentanyl reduces mesenteric blood flow.

131 Regarding the population of patients presenting for vascular surgery:

A Coronary artery disease is responsible for over 50% of the perioperative morbidity and mortality.
B The incidence of myocardial infarction following abdominal aneurysmectomy is 25–35%.
C The curve relating glomerular filtration rate to renal perfusion pressure is shifted to the left.
D Left ventricular ejection fraction of less than 50% is very rarely seen.
E Left ventricular compliance is only rarely reduced in this group.

128 A **True**   Its *S* isomer may be associated with fewer side
                      effects and equivalent anaesthetic effect.
     B **True**
     C **True**
     D **True**
     E **False**   Patients suffering emergence phenomena should be
                      nursed in a quiet environment and do not usually
                      require re-sedation.

129 A **True**   Body fat content can vary between 15% and 80%. In
                      the acute situation this compartment has little
                      relevance since its perfusion is so low.
     B **True**
     C **False**   It takes 4–5 times the elimination half-life.
     D **False**   The 95% CI of the ED_{95} of propofol is larger.
     E **False**   This is the case with volatile agents (isoflurane MAC
                      0.75% vs. 0.29%), but the MIR of propofol is not so
                      strongly affected (EC_{50} 8.1 vs. 5.4 $\mu g.ml^{-1}$).

130 A **True**   This is probably a centrally mediated compensation
                      for the fall in systemic pressure.
     B **False**   The fall is of the order of 20%.
     C **False**   It increases tone and increases splanchnic blood
                      flow by 20%.
     D **True**   It is several times more sensitive, and splanchnic
                      resistance rises approximately 10 times as fast.
     E **True**   Many drugs cause mesenteric flow to fall due to
                      their effect on blood pressure.

131 A **True**
     B **False**   It is 5–15%.
     C **False**   GFR is kept constant in the elevated range of these
                      patients' blood pressure.
     D **False**   It is seen in approximately a quarter of this
                      population.
     E **False**   It is usually reduced due to atherosclerosis, LV
                      hypertrophy and chronically elevated arterial
                      pressure.

132 **The following data are obtained from a 74-year-old female about to undergo pneumonectomy for small cell carcinoma: Na^+ 122 mmol.l⁻¹, K^+ 4.5 mmol.l⁻¹, urea 4.3 mmol.l⁻¹, glucose 4.3 mmol.l⁻¹, urine osmolality 480 mosm.l⁻¹.**

A She has renal failure.
B The urine osmolality is inappropriately high.
C This is consistent with ectopic secretion of ACTH or cortisol by the tumour.
D Water restriction may be an effective therapy.
E These abnormalities may have resulted from prolonged use of loop diuretics.

133 **Concerning tracheostomy:**

A It reduces serial respiratory deadspace.
B It should be performed via the first tracheal ring.
C It is safer using a percutaneous technique than using an open surgical technique.
D It is better tolerated by patients than orotracheal intubation.
E Use of a bevel-tipped tube reduces the risk of obstruction.

134 **$p < 0.05$ means that:**

A The sample groups came from different populations.
B The chance of a type 2 error is 5%.
C The power of the study is 95%.
D The study was successful.
E There is no need to repeat the study.

135 **Concerning thymoma:**

A It is usually malignant.
B It is usually diagnosed in association with myasthenia gravis.
C Thymectomy improves myasthenia gravis more if thymoma was present.
D It may cause stridor.
E Removal requires median sternotomy.

136 **Regarding tests for brain stem death:**

A They should be carried out on all patients from whom treatment is withdrawn on ITU.
B They examine all the cranial nerves except the olfactory.
C They must be repeated at least once.
D They require the presence of a neurologist or neurosurgeon.
E The presence of doll's eye movements indicates residual brain stem function.

132 A **False**   There is no evidence of this.
     B **False**   It is inappropriately low. Plasma osmolality is only
                      262 mosm.l^{-1}.
     C **False**   This would cause a Cushing's syndrome, with
                      sodium and water retention and hypokalaemia.
                      Plasma osmolality is usually normal.
     D **True**   This is the first-line treatment for the syndrome of
                      inappropriate ADH secretion, which is at the top of
                      the list of differential diagnoses.
     E **False**   Hypokalaemia would almost certainly be apparent.
                      In addition, urine osmolality would not be high
                      when serum osmolality was low.

133 A **True**
     B **False**   This should be avoided, since it renders the larynx
                      unstable.
     C **False**   There is no evidence to support this. The technique
                      is, however, time saving and simple.
     D **True**   This is the major advantage of tracheostomy in
                      weaning patients from mechanical ventilation.
     E **False**   Tubes are normally cut square to reduce the risk of
                      obstruction.

134 A **False**   It means that there is only a 5% or less chance that
                      they came from the same population.
     B **True**   A type 2 error occurs when the null hypothesis is
                      wrongly accepted (a difference is missed).
     C **False**   The power and the value of p are not directly
                      related.
     D **False**   Success and failure are determined by the
                      application of the results, not by the value of p.
     E **False**   See D.

135 A **False**
     B **True**
     C **False**   Removal of the thymus in the absence of a thymoma
                      seems to improve myasthenia more.
     D **True**   Oedema and haemorrhage may compress the larynx
                      or trachea.
     E **True**

136 A **False**   The majority of patients are not brain stem dead
                      when treatment is withdrawn on ITU.
     B **False**   The facial nerve (VII) is not tested.
     C **False**   They do not require repetition, although this is often
                      performed.
     D **False**   They require the presence of two doctors who have
                      been registered for 5 years or more.
     E **False**   This indicates lack of function.

137 Malignant hyperpyrexia:

A Always produces generalised muscle rigidity.
B Produces acidaemia and hypokalaemia.
C Is inherited as an autosomal dominant.
D Has a mortality well in excess of 50%.
E Is triggered by all anaesthetic vapours.

138 Depressed conscious level:

A May indicate hypovolaemia.
B Is a specific indicator of head injury.
C May be due to residual neuromuscular blockade.
D May be caused by hyperthermia and hypothermia.
E May coexist with an increased cerebral metabolic requirement for oxygen.

139 Regarding the physiological changes during exercise:

A Serum K^+ concentration increases.
B Cardiac output may rise to >20 l.min^{-1}.
C Left ventricular end-systolic volume may fall to 10 ml.
D Increases in minute volume and cardiac index do not occur until several seconds after exercise has started.
E An acidaemia develops.

140 Regarding electrical safety in the operating theatre:

A Connection through a person between the live terminal and earth will result in direct current flowing.
B As little as 20 mA of mains supply alternating current can cause ventricular fibrillation.
C Monitors connected to intracardiac catheters should not be earthed.
D Burns may occur at the site of the plate electrode during bipolar diathermy.
E Ohmic heating occurs at sites of high current density.

137 A **False** MH may occasionally present without the hallmark of rigidity and may occasionally affect only a few muscle groups such as the masseter.
B **False** It tends to produce acidaemia and hyperkalaemia.
C **True**
D **False** Once diagnosed, management with dantrolene, cooling and intensive support is generally successful as long as all triggering agents are removed.
E **False** It is not triggered by nitrous oxide, which is a vapour, but is triggered by all the halogenated volatile agents.

138 A **True** It occurs during severe hypovolaemia, when cerebral perfusion is impaired.
B **False** It has a variety of aetiologies.
C **False** Neuromuscular blocking agents do not cause a reduction in conscious level.
D **True** Either may cause a reduction in conscious level if severe enough.
E **True** The two may be related or independent. Seizures give rise to such a situation.

139 A **True** It may rise as high as 8 mmol.l^{-1} in the healthy adult with no apparent ill effects.
B **True** It may rise even higher in athletes.
C **False** It may fall to 20 ml.
D **False** There is pre-emption of exercise, and respiratory and cardiovascular 'responses' commence before the exercise begins.
E **True** This is mainly a lactic acidaemia, partially compensated by a respiratory alkalosis. It quickly resolves after exercise.

140 A **False** This will occur with alternating current, but not with direct current.
B **False** As little as 50 mA of mains supply AC may cause VF.
C **True** Otherwise, microshock may be caused. As little as 100 μA are required to cause VF.
D **False** A plate electrode is not required for bipolar diathermy.
E **True** Electrical current is concentrated and causes local heating. This is the principle of operation of medical diathermy.

141 Pneumothorax is possible with:

A Paravertebral block.
B Intercostal block.
C Stellate ganglion block.
D Brachial plexus block.
E Coeliac plexus block.

142 Carbon monoxide inhalation can cause hypoxia because:

A The affinity of carbon monoxide for oxygen binding sites on haemoglobin is 240 times greater than that of oxygen for the same sites.
B Oxygen delivery to the tissues is decreased.
C The oxyhaemoglobin dissociation curve is shifted to the left.
D 2,3-DPG is increased.
E There is an associated hypercapnia.

143 Regarding the applied anatomy of the spinal canal:

A The dura extends from foramen magnum to sacral hiatus.
B The spinal cord ends at L1/2 at birth.
C The conus medullaris is the tapered final limit of the cord.
D The cauda equina consists of spinal nerve routes below L1.
E The epidural space is between the dura and the bony and ligament walls of the spinal canal.

144 The most common complications of stellate ganglion block include:

A Horner's syndrome.
B Brachial plexus block.
C Local haematoma.
D Hoarseness of voice.
E Neuralgia around the chest wall.

145 Regarding drug administration during CPR:

A Central venous access is necessary for successful outcome.
B Intralingual or sublingual routes are acceptable alternatives if there is no venous access.
C The intra-arterial route should never be used.
D The dose for intra-osseus administration is 2–2.5 times more than that for i.v. administration.
E The dose for intratracheal administration is the same as that for i.v. administration.

141   A **True**
      B **True**
      C **True**
      D **True**
      E **True**

142   A **True**
      B **True**
      C **True**
      D **False**   The increase in 2,3-DPG is a late, compensatory
                     mechanism to increase oxygen release in the
                     tissues.
      E **False**   Hypoxia may stimulate hyperventilation, although
                     this is often absent. Hypocapnia is more often seen
                     than hypercapnia.

143   A **False**
      B **False**
      C **True**
      D **True**
      E **True**
The dura extends from the foramen magnum to S2. The spinal
canal at birth ends at L3. In adults it ends at L1/2.

144   A **True**
      B **False**
      C **True**
      D **True**
      E **False**
If the anaesthetic is injected into the paravertebral fascia, it can
spread along the fascial plane to involve the brachial plexus. This
complication is rare.

145   A **False**   Any venous route is acceptable to start with.
      B **False**   These routes have no role.
      C **False**   This can be used if this is the only one available.
      D **False**   It is same as that for the i.v. route.
      E **False**   It is 2–2.5 times more than that for the i.v. route.

146 The following increase the incidence of postoperative nausea and vomiting:

A Hypotension.
B Pain.
C Etomidate.
D Nitrous oxide.
E Female gender.

147 NSAIDs:

A Inhibit cyclooxygenase.
B May inhibit phosphodiesterase.
C Do not affect opioid requirement after laparotomy.
D Have irreversible effects on the renal vasculature.
E Do not affect gastric mucosa on parenteral administration.

148 Monitoring of the neuromuscular junction in a patient with signs of partial reversal of a non-depolarising neuromuscular block is likely to reveal:

A Characteristic absence of fade.
B Post-tetanic facilitation.
C Normal or decreased single twitch height.
D Train-of-four (TOF) ratio of <0.7.
E Decreased post-tetanic count (PTC).

149 The following cause a reduction in $CMRO_2$:

A Lignocaine.
B Barbiturates.
C Isoflurane.
D Enflurane.
E Suxamethonium.

150 The following preconditions must be met before considering the diagnosis of brain stem death:

A Sedatives and muscle relaxants must be excluded as causes for cessation of spontaneous breathing.
B Coma must not be due to primary hypothermia.
C The patient's condition is primarily due to extensive structural damage, metabolic derangement or serious endocrine insufficiency.
D The patient is not on a ventilator.
E Serum electrolytes and arterial blood gases are in the normal range.

146 A **True**
     B **True**
     C **True**
     D **True**
     E **True**
     Other factors include the use of narcotics, bowel surgery, gynaecological surgery, dehydration and ENT surgery.

147 A **True**
     B **True**   Especially indomethacin.
     C **False**   They are known to have an opioid sparing effect.
     D **False**   The effect is due to inhibition of prostaglandin synthesis that is reversible.
     E **False**   The gastric mucosa is affected due to reduction in the cytoprotective effect of gastric prostaglandins, and not due to local irritation.

148 A **False**   Features will be the same as those of partial block; fade should be present.
     B **True**
     C **True**
     D **True**   A patient with TOF > 0.7 is unlikely to show any sign of partial block.
     E **False**   PTC decreases only at very deep levels of neuromuscular block.

149 A **True**   Lignocaine in clinical doses reduces $CMRO_2$ and CBF.
     B **True**   All i.v. anaesthetics (with the exception of ketamine) reduce $CMRO_2$.
     C **True**   All volatile anaesthetics reduce $CMRO_2$ and isoflurane has more effect than others.
     D **True**
     E **False**   Suxamethonium does not cross the blood–brain barrier.

150 A **True**
     B **True**
     C **False**   Endocrine insufficiency and metabolic derangements can be reversible.
     D **False**   At the time of these tests patients are likely to be on a ventilator. As part of the brain stem tests the ventilator may have to be disconnected to ensure that the patient does not breathe spontaneously despite having the systemic carbon dioxide raised to above 6 kPa.
     E **True**

151   In a neonate (full term):

A Oxygen consumption is about twice that of an adult on a weight basis.

B Alveolar ventilation is about twice that of an adult on a weight basis.

C Carbon dioxide production is about twice that of an adult on a weight basis.

D Tidal volume is about the same as that of an adult on a weight basis.

E Functional residual capacity does not reach adult levels (30 ml/kg) until 6 months of age.

152   The recommended emergency measures in a child with suspected epiglottitis and presenting with respiratory distress are:

A Trial of aerosolised racemic adrenaline to prevent intubation of trachea.

B Indirect laryngoscopy or neck X-ray to confirm diagnosis.

C Preparation for emergency tracheal intubation and tracheostomy.

D Repeated measurement of $PaCO_2$ for early indication of physical exhaustion.

E Intravenous induction with thiopentone and suxamethonium to ensure quick intubation.

153   With caudal epidural block in children:

A Adequate pain relief is achieved after circumcision and anal operations.

B Pain relief after lower abdominal surgery cannot be achieved.

C Chances of dural puncture are higher than in adults.

D Use of morphine in the epidural space is contraindicated.

E More than 0.5 ml. kg^{-1} of 0.25% bupivacaine is contraindicated.

154   For perioperative myocardial ischaemia:

A Lead II gives indication about areas supplied by the right coronary artery.

B Precordial lead V5 will detect ischaemia in areas supplied by the left coronary artery.

C Combined monitoring of leads II and V5 will detect all ischaemic episodes.

D ST segment depression of 1 mm is a significant indicator.

E Transoesophageal echocardiography allows earlier detection than ECG changes.

151 A **True**
     B **True**
     C **True**
     D **True**   Relatively high oxygen consumption in a neonate results in similarly increased carbon dioxide production and increased alveolar ventilation. This is achieved by a proportionate increase in respiratory rate while the tidal volume (per kg) remains the same as that of an adult.
     E **False**   FRC reaches adult levels at about 4 days of age.

152 A **False**   This is recommended in croup, but not in epiglottitis.
     B **False**   Once epiglottitis is suspected, arrangements should be made on an urgent basis to secure tracheal intubation under inhalational anaesthesia with a back-up facility for emergency tracheostomy or cricothyrotomy. Time should not be wasted on confirming the diagnosis, especially if the child is in distress.
     C **True**
     D **False**   This may be more appropriate in croup.
     E **False**   Inhalational induction with halothane is recommended.

153 A **True**
     B **False**   It is an accepted method of analgesia after lower abdominal surgery.
     C **True**   The dural sac ends at S3 in the neonate and at S1 in an adult.
     D **False**   There is an increased incidence of apnoea and pruritus but it is not contraindicated.
     E **False**   Larger doses are used to block segments supplying the abdomen.

154 A **True**
     B **True**
     C **False**   Sensitivity of combined monitoring is 80%.
     D **True**
     E **True**   Segmental akinesia or dyskinesia are more sensitive signs of ischaemia.

155 In hypertrophic cardiomyopathy with outflow obstruction:

A Atrial fibrillation is poorly tolerated.
B Angina is relieved on assuming supine position.
C A modest degree of myocardial depression is acceptable during anaesthesia.
D Dopamine is the drug of choice to treat intraoperative hypotension.
E Use of a β-blocker is contraindicated.

156 In a patient with an artificial pacemaker:

A Hyperkalaemia can increase the stimulation threshold.
B Hypokalaemia can decrease the stimulation threshold.
C Arterial hypoxaemia does not alter the stimulation threshold.
D Thiopentone and halothane cause significant change in the stimulation threshold.
E Use of isoflurane is safe.

157 Regarding rate pressure product:

A It is a product of heart rate and mean arterial pressure.
B Between 5500 and 7000 is normal.
C More than 8000 reflects increased oxygen demand of myocardium.
D It is an excellent predictor of intraoperative myocardial ischaemia.
E It is as good as the Tripple index as a predictor of intraoperative myocardial ischaemia.

158 The following preoperative abnormalities suggest a high mortality after hepatobiliary surgery:

A Serum bilirubin more than 3 mg.dl^{-1}.
B Serum albumin below 3 g.dl^{-1}.
C Poorly controlled ascites.
D Encephalopathy.
E Prolonged prothrombin time.

159 The following can be used to prevent reperfusion injury:

A Allopurinol.
B Glutathione dismutase.
C Xanthine oxidase.
D Superoxide dismutase.
E Mannitol.

155 A **True**   Diastolic filling is impaired in these patients and its
                    dependence on atrial contraction is thus increased.
    B **True**   Presumably because the increase in ventricular size
                    during recumbency decreases the outflow
                    obstruction.
    C **True**   It is the increase in contractility that increases
                    obstruction.
    D **False**   Hypotension is due to vasodilatation ± outflow
                    obstruction. α agonists should be used and drugs
                    with β activity should be avoided. Fluids and
                    phenylephrine should be used as the first line of
                    treatment.
    E **False**   β-blockers reduce the outflow obstruction and
                    produce moderate bradycardia, which improves
                    diastolic filling.

156 A **False**   Stimulation threshold is decreased in hyperkalaemia
                    and increased in hypokalaemia.
    B **False**
    C **False**   Hypoxia, hypercarbia and catecholamines can
                    significantly affect the threshold.
    D **False**   Anaesthetics in general have little effect, although
                    halothane is itself arrhythmogenic.
    E **True**

157 A **False**   It is a product of heart rate and systolic blood
                    pressure.
    B **False**   Up to 12 000 is normal.
    C **False**   More than 15 000 should be avoided.
    D **False**   It is a poor predictor.
    E **True**   The Tripple index (RPP × PCWP) is as good as RPP.

158 A **True**
    B **True**
    C **True**
    D **True**
    E **True**

159 A **True**
    B **True**   A free radical scavenger.
    C **False**   A substrate for free radical production.
    D **True**   A free radical scavenger.
    E **True**   A free radical scavenger.

160 Among lung disorders:

A Alveolar compliance is reduced in pulmonary fibrosis.
B Airway resistance is increased in ARDS.
C FRC is increased in ARDS.
D Atelectasis increases shunt.
E Total lung capacity is increased in COPD.

160 A **True**
     B **False**   ARDS affects primarily the alveoli, causing reduced
                     compliance and FRC.
     C **False**   See above.
     D **True**   Ventilation is reduced in atelectatic lung.
     E **True**   Due to the hyperinflation caused by interstitial
                     destruction.

Paper 5

161 Regarding cardiovascular risk:

A Risk of repeat myocardial infarction is greatest in the first 3 months following infarction.

B Reinfarction is more likely in survivors of non-Q wave infarcts than in survivors of Q wave infarcts.

C All patients with angina should receive an exercise test or cardiac catheterisation preoperatively.

D Asymptomatic cardiac murmurs may be safely ignored.

E All arrhythmias, except sinus arrhythmia, are associated with increased perioperative risk.

162 Regarding preoperative preparation:

A Abstention from food and drink significantly elevates intragastric pH.

B Most preoperatively starved patients have an empty stomach.

C Intake of clear fluids up to 1 h before surgery has been shown to produce similar gastric contents to traditional starvation methods.

D The oral contraceptive pill must be stopped before surgery.

E All patients who are not adequately starved for anaesthesia should receive metoclopramide to speed gastric emptying.

163 In chronic renal failure:

A Myopathy, sensory and motor neuropathy and autonomic neuropathy are seen.

B The hypertension seen was usually present before renal failure commenced.

C A metabolic acidosis with a compensatory respiratory alkalosis is common.

D Platelet dysfunction is common.

E Hyperparathyroidism may cause hypocalcaemia.

Answers

161 A **True**
     B **True**
     C **False** This is excessively aggressive.
     D **False** All murmurs should be identified, and any associated risk quantified.
     E **True** Even premature atrial or ventricular beats are associated with increased risk.

162 A **False** It may lower pH.
     B **False** Very few patients will have an empty stomach, even after prolonged starvation.
     C **False** Drinking clear fluids up to 2 h before surgery.
     D **False** It should only be stopped before major surgery or in those at high risk of thrombosis.
     E **False**

163 A **True**
     B **False** Renal failure causes hypertension, although some cases of renal failure are due to hypertension.
     C **True** Due to failure of renal excretion of acid.
     D **True**
     E **False** The low calcium levels of renal failure cause secondary hyperparathyroidism.

164 Regarding antidepressants:

A Tricyclic antidepressants are negatively inotropic and proconvulsant.

B Tricyclic antidepressants potentiate indirect sympathomimetics but not exogenous catecholamines.

C Serotonin reuptake inhibitors cause a similar degree of anticholinergic side effects as do tricyclics.

D Monoamine oxidase inhibitors usually reduce blood pressure and cause postural hypotension.

E The majority of currently used monoamine oxidase inhibitors are selective MAOIs.

165 Regarding electrocardiogram (ECG) monitoring:

A The wide frequency response of ECG monitoring helps eliminate baseline drift and motion artefacts.

B Precordial leads are unipolar, while leads I, II and III are bipolar.

C The CM5 configuration is a useful monitor of anterior myocardial ischaemia.

D Leads II and MCL1 are appropriate leads for arrhythmia detection in a three-lead system.

E Lead V2 is the most sensitive single lead for detection of ischaemia.

166 Regarding capnography:

A Side-stream analysis suffers with a smaller lag than main-stream analysis.

B An increase in the end-tidal to arterial carbon dioxide gradient indicates an increase in anatomical deadspace fraction.

C End-tidal carbon dioxide tension may exceed arterial carbon dioxide tension.

D Most devices compare the absorption of monochromatic light in the patient sample to a reference sample.

E Errors are caused by absorption of light by water vapour and nitrous oxide.

167 The following signs are reliable gauges of the onset of anaesthesia:

A Loss of eyelash reflex.

B Loss of pupil reflex.

C Rate and depth of ventilation.

D Direction of gaze.

E Pattern of ventilation.

164 A **True**
     B **False** Indirect sympathomimetics have a reduced effect.
     C **False** Tricyclic agents have a greater anticholinergic effect.
     D **True**   They may cause hypertensive crises in combination
                  with indirect sympathomimetics.
     E **False** The majority of currently used MAOIs are non-
                  selective.

165 A **False** A narrow frequency response eliminates drift and
                  artefacts.
     B **True**
     C **True**   It is probably second only to V5 in detecting
                  myocardial ischaemia.
     D **True**
     E **False** Lead V5 is probably the best at detection.

166 A **False** The lag in side-stream analysis amounts to a few
                  seconds.
     B **False** It indicates a rise in the alveolar deadspace fraction.
     C **True**   If the inspired gas contains carbon dioxide or in a
                  dynamic situation where hyperventilation has
                  commenced.
     D **True**
     E **True**

167 A **False** This is predictable with barbiturates, but newer
                  agents (e.g. propofol) produce this unreliably.
     B **False** This is unreliable.
     C **False**
     D **False**
     E **True**   At first, there is variation in duration of each breath,
                  then expiration becomes active and then becomes
                  passive again.

168 Regarding the effects of i.v. induction agents on the cardiovascular system:

A Induction with propofol causes myocardial depression and vasodilatation.
B The fall in arterial pressure caused by induction with barbiturates is accompanied by a compensatory tachycardia.
C Midazolam causes less cardiovascular disturbance in inducing anaesthesia in healthy patients than thiopentone.
D Ketamine causes predominantly systolic hypertension.
E The cardiovascular effects of ketamine may be obtunded by pretreatment with midazolam.

169 Regarding intravenous anaesthesia:

A A closed loop system requires electroencephalographic input.
B Total i.v. anaesthesia provides better surgical conditions than volatile anaesthesia during bowel surgery.
C The major problem with total i.v. anaesthesia is the potential variability of response.
D Monitoring the depth of anaesthesia during i.v. maintenance is more difficult than during volatile maintenance.
E The existence of biophase lag during total i.v. anaesthesia increases the risk of awareness.

170 Regarding pulmonary function following abdominal surgery:

A The reduction in pulmonary function following abdominal surgery is due to a reduction in diaphragmatic and abdominal muscle function.
B Upper abdominal surgery decreases functional residual capacity by 30%.
C An infusion of doxapram increases postoperative arterial oxygen tension.
D An FEV_1 to FVC ratio of 0.55 is predictive of postoperative pulmonary problems.
E Opioid analgesia has little effect on the incidence of respiratory complications.

171 In patients with diabetes mellitus:

A Coronary lesions often require surgical repair.
B Silent myocardial ischaemia is more common than in other vascular patients.
C Healing after surgery is as good as in non-diabetic patients.
D Postoperative ventricular failure is more common.
E Homeostasis of arterial pressure is often impaired.

168 A **True**
     B **True**   This is not seen with propofol.
     C **False**   The fall in blood pressure is similar in both groups.
     D **True**   Typically, systolic pressure rises 20–40 mmHg, while
                    diastolic rises by less.
     E **True**

169 A **False**   The closed loop may use any information such as
                    blood pressure or respiratory rate. EEG data may
                    make the closed loop more reliable.
     B **True**   Nitrous oxide inflates the bowel.
     C **True**
     D **True**   Expired volatile agent concentration may be
                    measured in real time, but plasma agent
                    concentration cannot.
     E **True**

170 A **True**
     B **True**   This reduction may last for up to a week.
     C **True**   It reduces the hypoventilation commonly seen after
                    this type of surgery.
     D **True**   This indicates an element of obstructive lung
                    disease and correlates with the occurrence of
                    postoperative problems.
     E **False**   It causes hypoventilation, obstructive apnoea and
                    increased atelectasis.

171 A **False**   The lesions are often distal and cannot be repaired
                    surgically.
     B **True**   Autonomic neuropathy is the cause.
     C **False**   Healing is poor.
     D **True**   Insulin-dependent diabetes is an independent risk
                    factor.
     E **True**   Autonomic neuropathy often makes these patients
                    unstable after induction of anaesthesia.

172 **The following values were found in a young male vagrant admitted to the intensive therapy unit: Na$^+$ 133 mmol.l^{-1}, K$^+$ 4.2 mmol.l^{-1}, Cl$^-$ 98 mmol.l^{-1}, HCO$_3^-$ 9 mmol.l^{-1}, PaCO$_2$ 2.3 kPa. He gives a history of antifreeze ingestion.**

A He should be mechanically ventilated and his PaCO$_2$ normalised.
B He has an anion gap.
C Sodium bicarbonate is contraindicated.
D He should receive an alcohol infusion.
E Dialysis is of little use in this patient.

173 **Regarding the head-injured patient admitted to the intensive therapy unit:**

A Rapid, definitive care will reverse the primary injury to some degree.
B Reduction in central venous pressure always increases cerebral blood flow.
C Hyperventilation may increase blood flow to injured areas of the brain.
D A fall in PaO$_2$ from 13 kPa to 10 kPa will consistently cause an increase in intracranial pressure.
E A slight head-down tilt (5–10°) increases cerebral blood flow.

174 **Thyrotoxicosis:**

A May present as cardiac failure.
B May be treated acutely with corticosteroids.
C Causes an elevated VO$_2$.
D Is frequently caused by neoplasm.
E Results in hair loss and greasy skin.

175 **Open cardiac massage:**

A Is indicated in all traumatised patients not responding to closed chest massage.
B Is useful in an asystolic patient.
C Requires thoracotomy.
D Is more effective than closed chest cardiac massage.
E Should pause during mechanical inspiration.

172 A **False**   His $PaCO_2$ is appropriately low to compensate for his marked metabolic acidosis.

  B **True**   The sum of anions does not equal that of cations. Other negatively charged molecules account for the gap.

  C **False**   He has a very severe metabolic acidosis due to the metabolites of the ethylene glycol and will benefit from sodium bicarbonate.

  D **True**   This saturates the breakdown pathway of ethylene glycol and slows the formation of its harmful metabolites.

  E **False**   Dialysis should be established since ethylene glycol is widely distributed and slowly excreted via the kidney.

173 A **False**   The primary injury consists of irreversible brain damage. The aim of management is to prevent secondary injury.

  B **False**   If ICP exceeds CVP then further reductions may not increase CBF.

  C **True**   Hypocarbia reduces cerebral blood volume and thus ICP. The unresponsive, injured part of the brain may thus enjoy increased blood flow.

  D **False**   ICP only starts to rise when PaO_2 falls to 8 kPa or below.

  E **False**   This causes cerebral oedema and a rise in venous pressure, and may result in an overall reduction in CBF.

174 A **True**   High-output cardiac failure.

  B **True**   These may be effective in the acute phase in combination with β-blockers, although it may be several hours before they begin to have a noticeable effect.

  C **True**   Metabolic rate may rise dramatically, increasing water and calorie requirements.

  D **False**   Thyroid tumours rarely secrete excessive quantities of thyroxine.

  E **False**   Hypothyroidism typically produces these signs.

175 A **False**   It is seldom effective when closed massage is not. If the patient already has a thoracotomy or laparotomy, it is justified.

  B **False**   There is no evidence of its efficacy in this situation.

  C **False**   It may be performed via laparotomy.

  D **True**   Cardiac output is higher using open massage, but it is questionable if survival is better.

  E **False**   There is no need for this.

176 Regarding tracheostomy:

  A It often helps in weaning patients from mechanical ventilation.
  B It carries the risk of pneumothorax.
  C It reduces physiological deadspace.
  D It may give rise to tracheal stenosis.
  E Transcutaneous tracheostomy should always be performed via the cricothyroid membrane.

177 Regarding the anaesthetic management of a patient undergoing thymectomy for myasthenia gravis:

  A Anticholinesterase therapy should be changed to neostigmine 1 week prior to surgery.
  B Omission of the anticholinesterase on the morning of surgery is dangerous.
  C The ITU should be informed.
  D Suxamethonium produces a prolonged and dense block.
  E If a muscle relaxant is needed, atracurium must be used.

178 Concerning local anaesthetic toxicity:

  A It may occur after administration of small doses of local anaesthetics.
  B It is related to the site of administration.
  C It is more likely if administration is rapid.
  D It causes CNS effects before cardiovascular effects.
  E The cardiovascular collapse to CNS symptoms concentration ratio is higher for bupivacaine than lignocaine.

179 Ascent to 10 000 m above sea level will induce:

  A A reduction in pulmonary deadspace fraction.
  B An increase in red cell 2,3-diphosphoglycerate concentration.
  C Anaemia.
  D Renal conservation of bicarbonate.
  E Pulmonary oedema in 1% of people.

176 A **True**   The major effect is probably in making the airway more tolerable.
     B **True**
     C **True**   Although the reduction is small and probably not a major part of the effect on the patient.
     D **True**   Scarring after removal of the tracheostomy may result in stenosis.
     E **False**

177 A **False**   There is no need to change to neostigmine.
     B **False**   Management of muscle weakness during anaesthesia is neither difficult nor dangerous. The patient should be managed on intensive care after the operation, when anticholinesterase therapy may be reintroduced.
     C **True**   See above.
     D **False**   The myasthenic patient may be resistant to suxamethonium.
     E **False**   If muscle relaxation is required, any short- to medium-acting agent is appropriate. The advantage of atracurium in not requiring the liver or kidneys for its elimination is not of particular importance in the myasthenic.

178 A **True**   Administration of only 1 ml into the vertebral artery may cause CNS toxicity.
     B **True**   Certain sites have a much more rapid uptake than others, resulting in higher plasma levels and greater toxicity for a given dose.
     C **True**   This is especially true if administration is into a vein or artery.
     D **True**   CNS toxicity occurs typically with much lower plasma levels than are required to produce CVS toxicity. This difference is not so wide in the case of bupivacaine.
     E **False**   It is lower – see D .

179 A **False**   This does not occur.
     B **True**   This increases oxygen availability to the tissues and occurs over several days at altitude.
     C **False**   An increase in haemoglobin concentration may occur.
     D **False**   There is renal compensation for the respiratory alkalosis, and consequent urinary loss of bicarbonate.
     E **True**

180 Regarding epidural anaesthesia:

A It always causes some degree of sympathetic blockade.
B It is contraindicated when the platelet count is below 100×10^9 platelets.l^{-1}.
C It should not be performed below the L5/S1 junction.
D It increases left ventricular stroke work index.
E Epidural opioids should be used at approximately 10% of the dose used systemically for analgesia.

181 In stored blood there is an excess of:

A Ammonia.
B Hydrogen ions.
C Potassium ions.
D Calcium ions.
E 2,3-DPG.

182 During hypothermia:

A Solubility of carbon dioxide and oxygen is increased.
B Blood viscosity is increased.
C MAC is decreased.
D Renal blood flow is increased.
E Cerebral metabolism remains unaffected.

183 With regard to dermatomes:

A C1 has no dermal distribution.
B C8 is most distally distributed to the middle finger.
C T10 is at the level of the umbilicus.
D C7 supplies the thumb.
E L5 supplies the plantar surface of the heel of the foot.

184 Complications of coeliac plexus block include:

A Intravenous injection.
B Renal damage.
C Pneumothorax.
D Intra-arterial injection.
E Cauda equina syndrome.

180 A **False** The sympathetic outflow is from T1 to L2. Blockade confined to outflow above or below this will not cause sympatholysis.

B **False** There is no increased risk of an epidural haematoma.

C **False** Caudal epidural anaesthesia may be performed, with local anaesthetic being injected at the sacral hiatus.

D **False** LVSWI is reduced because the SVR ± contractility are reduced.

E **False** The dose used depends upon which opioid is used. Factors such as tissue binding, lipid solubility and potency are important.

181 A **True**
B **True**
C **True**
D **False**
E **False**
Stored blood is low in calcium ions and 2,3-DPG.

182 A **True**
B **True**
C **True**
D **False**
E **False** $CMRO_2$ falls by 6–8% for each 1°C fall in temperature.
The kidney has the largest proportionate reduction in blood of all the major organs. Both glomerular filtration rate and renal plasma flow are decreased.

183 A **True**
B **False**
C **True**
D **False**
E **False**
C7 is the most distally distributed dermatome to the middle finger in the upper extremity. The thumb is supplied by C6 and the little finger by C8. S1 supplies the plantar surface of the heel of the foot.

184 A **True**
B **True**
C **True**
D **True**
E **False**
Cauda equina syndrome is a recognised complication of subarachnoid block. It is neither reported nor conceivable with the coeliac plexus block.

185 **The following factors increase the incidence of perioperative morbidity associated with day-case surgery:**

A Prolonged surgery.
B General anaesthesia as compared to local anaesthesia.
C Hypertension.
D Chronic lung disease.
E Age more than 55 years.

186 **The following surgical procedures warrant increased use of anti-emetic treatment:**

A Upper abdominal surgery.
B Knee arthroscopy.
C Laparoscopy.
D Strabismus surgery.
E Orchidopexy.

187 **Risk factors of developing acute renal failure after NSAIDs include:**

A Old age.
B Paediatric age group.
C Pre-existing renal disease.
D Hypertension.
E Diabetes.

188 **Regarding recovery of muscles from non-depolarising neuromuscular block:**

A Adequate tidal volume ensures complete recovery of the respiratory muscles.
B Head lift sustained for >5 s ensures adequate recovery of the respiratory muscles.
C Vocal cords recover earlier than eye muscles.
D Patients able to oxygenate themselves have a TOF ratio of >0.7.
E Ability to open the eyes does not guarantee lack of diplopia.

189 **Isoelectric EEG:**

A Associated with barbiturates implies no metabolic activity in the brain cells.
B With barbiturates causes a decrease in $CMRO_2$ to about 5–10% of normal.
C With isoflurane offers cerebral protection.
D Is a typical feature of narcotic overdose.
E Can be seen with 2 MAC of isoflurane.

185   A **True**
      B **True**
      C **True**
      D **True**
      E **False**   Only extremes of age increase the risk.

186   A **True**
      B **False**   Peripheral surgery is associated with increased risk
                      of neither nausea nor vomiting.
      C **True**
      D **True**
      E **True**

187   A **True**
      B **False**   This is not a risk factor.
      C **True**
      D **True**
      E **True**

188   A **False**   Tidal volume can be maintained despite muscle
                      weakness.
      B **True**
      C **True**
      D **False**   See A.
      E **True**   Extraocular muscles are more sensitive than
                      obicularis oculi.

189   A **False**   Some activity remains to preserve the cellular
                      integrity.
      B **False** $CMRO_2$ is reduced to about 40% of normal.
      C **True**
      D **False**   Narcotics have a minimal effect.
      E **True**

190   Diagnostic tests to confirm brain stem death should ensure:

A Lack of corneal reflex.
B Fixed and dilated pupils.
C Absent vestibulo-ocular reflexes.
D Absent gag reflex.
E Absent spinal reflexes.

191   Regarding retinopathy of prematurity:

A The most significant risk factor is prematurity.
B It is seen only in infants receiving supplemental oxygen.
C Infants born at 38 weeks' gestation are not at risk.
D 80% of the retinal changes regress spontaneously.
E Monitoring of oxygen tension in the umbilical artery should prevent the risk.

192   In inspiratory stridor developing 6 h after rigid bronchoscopy in a 6-year-old child:

A The most likely cause is extrathoracic upper airway oedema.
B Complete respiratory obstruction is imminent.
C Aerosolised racemic adrenaline has no therapeutic value.
D Endotracheal intubation must be performed.
E Dexamethasone will definitely reduce oedema once the airway is secured.

193   Risk factors for the development of ischaemic heart disease are:

A Male gender.
B Hypercholesterolaemia.
C Hypertension.
D Cigarette smoking.
E Diabetes mellitus.

194   The following indicate myocardial ischaemia on transoesophageal echocardiography:

A Hypokinesia of left ventricular wall.
B Dyskinesia of ventricular wall.
C Impaired systolic thickening of myocardium.
D Impaired diastolic relaxation of myocardium.
E Increased left ventricular end-diastolic volume.

190   A **True**
       B **True**
       C **True**
       D **True**
       E **False**   Spinal reflexes may be present despite diagnosed
                       brain stem death.

191   A **True**
       B **False**   Retinopathy has been seen in infants who did not
                       receive supplemental oxygen.
       C **False**   Risk continues up to 44 weeks of gestation age.
       D **True**
       E **False**   Monitoring of a preductal (i.e. right radial) artery is
                       desirable.

192   A **True**   Intrathoracic airway obstruction is more likely to
                       produce expiratory stridor.
       B **False**   Although it is a risk.
       C **False**   In most cases aerosolised adrenaline and humidified
                       oxygen should suffice and endotracheal intubation is
                       required only if these measures fail and obstruction
                       worsens.
       D **False**   This is indicated only if other methods fail.
       E **False**   Although frequently used, efficacy of
                       dexamethasone is undocumented.

193   A **True**
       B **True**
       C **True**
       D **True**
       E **True**

194   A **True**
       B **True**
       C **True**
       D **True**
       E **False**   This indicates ventricular preload.

195 **The following will increase outflow obstruction associated with hypertrophic cardiomyopathy:**

   A β-stimulation.
   B α-stimulation.
   C Vasodilatation.
   D Volatile anaesthetic agents.
   E Digitalis.

196 **Failure of the heart to capture a temporary pacemaker's stimulus can occur with:**

   A Mechanical ventilation.
   B Cardioversion.
   C Propofol anaesthesia.
   D Central line placement.
   E Electrocautery.

197 **Indications for preoperative placement of a pacemaker include:**

   A RBBB.
   B LBBB.
   C Bifascicular heart block even without symptoms.
   D Bifascicular heart block with first-degree heart block.
   E Third-degree heart block.

198 **Regarding glomerular filtration:**

   A 180 litres of fluid are filtered each day.
   B Substances of molecular weight < 60 000 pass through the glomerular membrane easily.
   C Filtration is largely energy dependent.
   D Filtration rate (GFR) is reduced during hepatorenal syndrome.
   E GFR is markedly increased following frusemide.

199 **The following are known for their free-radical scavenging properties:**

   A Hydrogen peroxide.
   B Catalase.
   C Thiopentone.
   D Halothane.
   E Dimethylsulphoxide.

195 A **True**   Increased myocardial contractility increases the
                    outflow obstruction.
     B **False**   Increased afterload reduces the obstruction.
     C **True**   Reducing end-diastolic ventricular size, precipitating
                    obstruction.
     D **False**   Modest decrease in contractility is beneficial.
     E **True**

196 A **True**   The common cause for failure to capture is
                    disconnection of electrode from the myocardium.
     B **True**
     C **False**
     D **True**
     E **False**

197 A **False**   Progression of isolated RBBB or LBBB to complete
                    heart block is very rare.
     B **False**
     C **False**   It may be indicated in symptomatic bifascicular
                    block.
     D **True**   This type of block has a high incidence of
                    progressing into complete heart block.
     E **True**

198 A **True**
     B **False**   Substances of molecular weight < 15 000 pass
                    through easily; those with molecular weight up to
                    40 000 pass if they are neutrally charged. Larger
                    molecules are not filtered.
     C **False**   Filtration depends on the balance between
                    hydrostatic and oncotic forces.
     D **True**
     E **False**   Frusemide has little effect on GFR.

199 A **False**   This may increase the level of superoxide radicals.
     B **True**
     C **True**
     D **False**   Inhalational agents are not known to have
                    free-radical scavenging properties.
     E **True**

200 **The following cause an increase in the pulmonary diffusing capacity:**

A Larger body surface area.
B Supine position.
C Polycythaemia.
D Low cardiac output.
E Chronic bronchitis.

200 A **True**   Bigger lungs have a bigger capacity.
     B **False**   This reduces it.
     C **True**   Anaemia reduces the capacity.
     D **False**
     E **False**   Airway disease has no effect unless alveoli are
                     affected.

Paper 6

201 Regarding hypertension:

A It is associated with aetiological factors other than atherosclerosis in approximately 10% of cases.

B It increases the risk of stroke, myocardial infarction and renal failure postoperatively.

C It may settle in anxious patients newly admitted to hospital.

D It should be managed intraoperatively by lowering blood pressure to normotensive levels.

E Diastolic hypertension is associated with much greater risk than systolic hypertension.

202 The following are risk factors for ischaemic heart disease:

A Weight gain.

B Hypertriglyceridaemia.

C Regular heavy exercise.

D Consumption of marijuana.

E Family history of ischaemic heart disease.

203 Regarding myotonic dystrophy:

A It is inherited in a dominant fashion and onset is during childhood.

B Endocrine disorders are common in conjunction with myotonic dystrophy.

C Cardiomyopathy and conduction defects are common.

D The response to non-depolarising muscle relaxants is usually normal.

E Suxamethonium should be used in reduced doses because of the possibility of prolonged muscle contraction.

204 Antipsychotic drugs:

A Have an anti-emetic action at the chemoreceptor trigger zone.

B Produce elation in the absence of psychosis.

C Block acetylcholine, dopamine, histamine and α_1 receptors.

D Have a mild anticonvulsant effect.

E May give rise to the neuroleptic malignant syndrome, a central disorder leading to pyrexia and muscle rigidity.

Answers

---

201 A **True**   Such as renal artery stenosis, endocrine disease or pregnancy.

   B **True**

   C **True**   Blood pressure must be re-measured in the anxious, hypertensive patient.

   D **False** This may lead to inadequate organ perfusion due to right shifting of autoregulation curves.

   E **False** There is no evidence of this.

202 A **True**   The risk from this is almost as great as that from smoking.

   B **False** Hypotriglyceridaemia is a risk factor.

   C **False**

   D **False** Alone, this is not a risk factor, although when combined with tobacco consumption relative risk rises.

   E **True**

203 A **False** Onset is often during the fourth decade.

   B **True**   Diabetes mellitus, hypothyroidism and adrenal insufficiency are common.

   C **True**   A pacemaker may be required.

   D **True**   Small doses are indicated in those patients with respiratory muscle weakness.

   E **False** Suxamethonium should not be used. Prolonged contraction may prevent ventilation.

204 A **True**   This is the basis of current use of phenothiazines as anti-emetics.

   B **False** The antipsychotics are mood-flatteners.

   C **True**   Their antagonism is mild at each of these receptors, but side effects and interactions are widespread.

   D **False** They are proconvulsant.

   E **True**   As in malignant hyperpyrexia, dantrolene is useful.

205 Regarding non-invasive arterial blood pressure measurement:

A The majority of automated devices use the 'oscillotonometric' method.

B Too small a cuff will cause falsely high readings.

C Most methods estimate both systolic and diastolic pressures once mean pressure is measured.

D Non-invasive measurement of the arterial pressure waveform is available in real time.

E Blood pressure may be correlated to the delay in pulse wave propagation between forehead and finger.

206 Volatile anaesthetic agents may be measured:

A In the operating theatre using portable mass spectrometry.

B Using a mass spectrometer with a response time of 1–3 ms.

C Using polychromatic infrared spectrometry without requiring agent preselection.

D Using mass spectrometry provided they have different molecular weights.

E Using a multi-potential vacuum electrode.

207 Regarding i.v. induction of anaesthesia:

A Intravenous induction speed is increased if lipophilic agents are used.

B Duration of effect is related to the speed of metabolism of the drug.

C Recovery after a single dose of i.v. induction agent to normal performance in a critical flicker fusion test depends upon the drug's clearance.

D Recovery from a single dose of i.v. induction agent is slower during hypovolaemia.

E The majority of i.v. induction agents are heavily plasma protein bound.

208 Regarding the effects of i.v. induction agents on cerebral haemodynamics:

A Thiopentone reduces CSF formation.

B Etomidate increases cerebral vascular resistance.

C Propofol does not affect cerebral vascular carbon dioxide reactivity.

D Thiopentone is a suitable agent for use during somatosensory evoked potential monitoring.

E Thiopentone protects the brain against ischaemic damage during transient hypotension.

205 A **False**   The majority use the oscillometric method.
     B **True**   Too wide a cuff will cause low readings.
     C **True**   Mean pressure is represented by the point of maximal oscillation.
     D **True**   The Finapres allows recording of a waveform.
     E **True**   This non-invasive method of blood pressure measurement is being developed.

206 A **True**
     B **False**   The response time is approximately 100–200 ms.
     C **True**   Multiple wavelengths allow identification of multiple agents.
     D **False**   If the relative molecular weights are the same, the products of ionisation are measured.
     E **False**   Such a device does not exist.

207 A **True**
     B **False**   Redistribution terminates action.
     C **True**   This takes longer than waking, and is dependent upon elimination of the drug from the body.
     D **True**   Elimination of the redistributed drug is delayed by poor compartmental perfusion.
     E **False**

208 A **True**   So do midazolam and etomidate.
     B **True**   By reducing cerebral metabolic rate.
     C **True**   In contrast to other agents.
     D **True**   Thiopentone does, however, cause a change in brain stem and cortical auditory evoked responses.
     E **True**   It is used for this purpose in neuroanaesthesia.

209 Regarding opioids:

A 66% nitrous oxide and pethidine 50–60 mg.h^{-1} has been widely used as an anaesthetic regime.
B Modest doses of opioid with 66% nitrous oxide in oxygen results in awareness in 1–2% of cases.
C Opioids block the metabolic response to surgery more effectively than local anaesthetics.
D An analgesic dose of morphine reduces the alveolar concentration required of isoflurane for anaesthesia by approximately 50%.
E Opioids are effective in producing amnesia.

210 The following occur as a result of the stress response to surgery:

A Increased production of adrenocorticotrophic hormone.
B Increased serum aldosterone levels.
C Increased blood glucose levels.
D Loss of up to 500 g of muscle protein.
E Increased tissue insensitivity to insulin.

211 Regarding the resting 12-lead ECG before vascular surgery:

A A normal ECG is not a useful predictor of low risk for postoperative ischaemia.
B ST segment depression in the resting ECG is not usually indicative of pathology.
C Unifocal ventricular ectopics do not indicate increased risk.
D Widespread ST segment depression may indicate ventricular aneurysm.
E Low voltage complexes may indicate pericardial effusion.

212 Concerning hypokalaemia:

A It is occasionally caused by lack of potassium-retaining hormone.
B It occurs as part of the stress response to injury.
C It may arise as a natural compensation during respiratory acidosis.
D It causes peakedT waves and U waves on the ECG.
E Arrhythmias may be managed temporarily with i.v. calcium chloride.

209 A **True**   Although this is not widely used now (see next
                       question).
     B **True**
     C **False**
     D **False**   Very large doses are required to attain this, although
                       such a decrease has never been demonstrated in
                       humans.
     E **False**   Volatile agents, i.v. agents and benzodiazepines
                       produce amnesia, but very large doses are required
                       to produce any amnesia with opioids.

210 A **True**
     B **True**
     C **True**
     D **True**
     E **False**   There is resistance to the effects of insulin.

211 A **False**   It is a good predictor. Only 8% of patients with a
                       normal ECG get postoperative ischaemia.
     B **False**   ST segment depression in two or more leads in the
                       resting ECG is associated with ischaemia in 50% of
                       patients postoperatively.
     C **False**   Risk is increased.
     D **False**   Persistent ST elevation after a myocardial infarction
                       is much more common.
     E **True**   Although this is relatively uncommon in the
                       asymptomatic patient presenting for vascular
                       surgery.

212 A **False**   There is no known potassium-retaining hormone.
     B **True**   Elevated levels of cortisol and aldosterone are
                       responsible.
     C **False**   It may be precipitated by respiratory or metabolic
                       alkalosis since renal potassium excretion is
                       reciprocal with proton excretion.
     D **False**   Hyperkalaemia causes peaked T waves.
     E **False**   Calcium chloride will exacerbate hypokalaemia-
                       induced arrhythmias.

213 Regarding fulminant hepatic failure:

A The most common cause is paracetamol hepatotoxicity.
B It may follow halothane anaesthesia.
C It is not caused by alcohol.
D It may occur after prolonged liver disease.
E Survival usually involves recovery to a state of chronic liver impairment.

214 Melaena:

A Results from colonic bleeding.
B May cause acute hypovolaemia.
C May be the only symptom of oesophageal varices.
D Causes a rapid deterioration in conscious level.
E Responds to administration of vasopressin.

215 Thoracostomy tubes:

A Require a trocar for their insertion.
B Should be inserted via an existing penetrating chest wound when draining a traumatic haemothorax.
C Should be clamped when transferring a patient.
D Should be inserted in the 6th intercostal space in the anterior axillary line.
E May be used to provide interpleural analgesia.

216 Decontamination of the digestive tract:

A Must be performed in patients with extensive burns.
B Reduces the risk of nosocomial pneumonia.
C Requires enteral administration of antibiotics.
D May be achieved by i.v. administration of antibiotics.
E Reduces translocation of bacteria from the gut to the bloodstream.

213 A **True**   Accounting for 48% of cases. Viral hepatitis accounts for 37% of cases.
    B **True**   The incidence is higher in females, the obese and following multiple exposures.
    C **False**   FHF can be caused by alcohol.
    D **False**   By definition, FHF does not follow prolonged liver disease.
    E **False**   Recovery, which occurs in approximately 50%, is usually complete.

214 A **False**   Melaena contains altered blood, which must be derived from the small intestine.
    B **True**
    C **True**   Other symptoms, such as haematemesis, may be absent, especially if the varices are small.
    D **True**   It may cause hypovolaemia.
    E **True**   Vasopressin elevates the blood pressure and constricts the gut vasculature.

215 A **False**   The trocar is potentially very dangerous and may puncture virtually any organ in the thorax or abdomen. Once an opening is made into the pleural space, forceps may be used to guide the tube in.
    B **False**   The tube may follow the line of the penetrating injury into organs such as lungs or liver. It is better to site a new drain between the mid-axillary line and the lateral edge of the pectoralis major.
    C **False**   Tension pneumothorax or haemothorax may develop.
    D **False**   This is too low, see B. In the anterior axillary line, the 2nd, 3rd or 4th spaces are ideal.
    E **True**   A patient with rib fractures often benefits from instillation of 50 ml 0.125% bupivacaine via the chest drain. The analgesia may be dependent upon the patient's position.

216 A **False**   It may occasionally be helpful, but is not mandatory.
    B **True**
    C **True**   Parenteral administration does not allow gut penetration.
    D **False**   See C.
    E **True**   Because most of the gut bacteria have been killed.

217 The following are true of brachial plexus block using the axillary approach:

A Sensory blockade over the C5 dermatome is reliable.
B The risk of pneumothorax is very low.
C 10 ml of local anaesthetic usually results in a good block.
D Bilateral blocks may be used.
E Systemic uptake is slower than from an intercostal block.

218 Immediate management of major anaphylaxis should include:

A Subcutaneous administration of adrenaline 1 mg.
B Infusion of at least 500 ml of colloid solution.
C Administration of 30% oxygen.
D Blood sampling for markers of hypersensitivity.
E Intubation and ventilation.

219 Pulse pressure:

A Increases in early hypovolaemic shock.
B Is increased by increasing heart rate.
C Is reduced if arterial compliance is reduced.
D Is overestimated in a damped pressure transduction system.
E Is increased by hypercapnia.

217 A **False**   Blockade from C6/7 to T2 is reliable. Higher blocks require larger volumes of local anaesthetic, catheter techniques or supplementation with other brachial plexus blocks or local infiltration.

B **True**   The medial wall of the axilla is several centimetres from the pleura.

C **False**   20–50 ml is required.

D **True**   This is acceptable because of the low risk of pneumothorax (unlike bilateral interscalene blocks). Care must be taken with the total dose of local anaesthetic.

E **True**   Plasma levels for a given dose of local anaesthetic are lower, presumably because of lower local blood flow.

218 A **False**   Major anaphylaxis (CVS collapse with other symptoms) should be treated with i.v. adrenaline (epinephrine).

B **False**   Crystalloids may be a better choice since they have no risk of anaphylactic response.

C **False**   100% oxygen must be administered.

D **False**   This is not part of the immediate management.

E **False**   The patient may not require intubation and ventilation.

219 A **False**   It is reduced due to vasoconstriction, reducing diastolic run-off.

B **False**   Increases in heart rate reduce the time available for diastolic run-off, increasing diastolic pressure.

C **False**   Non-compliant arteries increase systolic pressure.

D **False**   Damped systems tend to bring the apparent systolic and diastolic pressures towards the mean pressure, thus reducing the apparent pulse pressure.

E **True**   Hypercapnia tends to reduce diastolic pressure through vasodilatation and increase systolic pressure through the inotropic effect of elevated circulating catecholamine levels.

220 Apnoea (at residual volume) in the normal subject:

A Causes a rise in $PaCO_2$ of approximately 0.4–0.7 kPa.min^{-1}.
B For 8 min following 10 min of breathing 100% oxygen will cause hypoxaemia.
C Causes a fall in serum bicarbonate concentration.
D Is unlikely to cause serum pH to fall below 7.3.
E Causes pupillary dilatation.

221 Acute pancreatitis is complicated by:

A Fluid deficit.
B Hypercalcaemia.
C Hyperglycaemia.
D Pleural effusion.
E ARDS.

222 Advanced kyphoscoliosis leads to:

A Polycythaemia.
B Right ventricular enlargement.
C Decreased tidal volume.
D Obstructive lung disease.
E Increased deadspace to tidal volume ratio.

223 With regard to the myotomes of the upper limb:

A C5 is associated with flexion of shoulder.
B C8 &T1 extend the shoulder.
C Abduction and adduction of digits are affected by C7 & C8.
D Flexion and extension of digits are affected by C7 & C8.
E The wrist is moved by C6 & C7.

220 A **True**   The addition of the VCO_2 (e.g. 200 ml.min^{-1}) to the
                   cardiac output (e.g. 5 l.min^{-1}) causes a rise of PCO_2
                   from 5.3 kPa to 6.1 kPa. Addition of the VCO_2 for
                   1 min (200 ml) to the blood volume (5 l) will raise
                   $PaCO_2$ and $PvCO_2$ by approximately the same
                   amount, although there will be some absorption by
                   the tissues, reducing the increase.
     B **False**   The residual volume is approximately 40 ml.kg^{-1},
                   containing oxygen. 8 min of apnoea will consume
                   approximately 2 l of oxygen and produce 1.5 l of
                   carbon dioxide. The alveoli would thus contain
                   approximately 40% oxygen.
     C **False**   Accumulation of carbon dioxide causes a rise in
                   bicarbonate.
     D **False**   Serum pH will fall below 7.2.
     E **True**   The rise in carbon dioxide will cause an increase in
                   serum catecholamines.

221 A **True**
     B **False**   Hypocalcaemia is more likely.
     C **True**   Caused by low circulating insulin levels.
     D **True**   Caused by transdiaphragmatic irritation.
     E **True**

222 A **True**   Hypoxic stimulation of erythropoeisis.
     B **True**   Due to increased pulmonary vascular resistance
                   secondary to chronic restrictive lung disease.
     C **True**
     D **False**   Mainly restrictive lung disease.
     E **True**

223 A **True**
     B **False**
     C **False**
     D **True**
     E **True**
The shoulder is flexed by C5 and is extended by C6/C7/C8. The
elbow is flexed by C5/C6 and is extended by C7/C8. The wrist is
flexed and extended by C6/C7. The digits are flexed and extended
by C7/C8 and are abducted and adducted by T1.

224 Contraindication of the stellate ganglion block includes:

    A Second-degree heart block.
    B Recent myocardial infarction.
    C Reflex dystrophy.
    D Contralateral pneumothorax.
    E Contralateral diaphragmatic paralysis.

225 In the preoperative assessment of patients scheduled for day-case surgery:

    A ASA class 3 indicates mild systemic disease that is not incapacitating.
    B ASA class 3 patients carry the same risk of perioperative morbidity as ASA class 2.
    C Full blood count should be routinely performed on all patients.
    D ECG should be performed on everyone over 50 years of age.
    E Electrolytes should be investigated routinely.

226 Recognised consequences of inadequate pain relief after upper abdominal surgery include:

    A Decreased functional residual capacity.
    B Ileus.
    C Deep vein thrombosis.
    D Sodium and water retention.
    E Reduced systemic vascular resistance.

227 Reduced platelet adhesion following NSAIDs:

    A Is due to inhibition of thromboxane A_2 synthesis.
    B Is due to inhibition of factors VIII, X and XI.
    C Is of concern while epidural technique is being considered.
    D Causes insignificant changes in the bleeding time.
    E Can be reversed to normal within 24 h after discontinuation.

228 Characteristic haemodynamic changes in a patient at the early stage of systemic inflammatory response syndrome (SIRS) include:

    A Increased cardiac output.
    B Reduced systemic vascular resistance (SVR).
    C Hypertension and tachycardia.
    D Hypoperfusion of vital organs.
    E Increased filling pressures.

224 A **True**
     B **True**
     C **False**   Stellate ganglion block is indicated in the treatment
                      of this condition.
     D **True**
     E **True**
Reflex dystrophy is one of the indications for a stellate ganglion
block. Other indications include acute herpes zoster,
hyperhydrosis, vascular spasm or thrombosis in the head and
upper extremity area.

225 A **False**   ASA class 3 indicates severe systemic disease that is
                      not incapacitating.
     B **False**   The risk is higher.
     C **False**   Only adult females or males over 50 years of age.
     D **True**   This is controversial.
     E **False**   Patients over 70 years of age or those taking
                      diuretics or digitalis.

226 A **True**   Due to diaphragmatic splinting.
     B **True**
     C **True**   Due to delayed and reduced mobility.
     D **True**   Secondary to aldosterone release as a part of the
                      stress phenomenon.
     E **False**   Catecholamine release due to stress causes
                      vasoconstriction.

227 A **True**
     B **False**
     C **True**   Although confirmatory evidence is lacking.
     D **False**   Prolongation in bleeding time is significant.
     E **False**   Can take up to a few days.

228 A **True**   Reduced SVR causes increased cardiac ouput.
     B **True**
     C **False**   Hypotension is characteristic.
     D **True**
     E **False**   Filling pressures are decreased due to
                      vasodilatation.

229 A rise in intracranial pressure (ICP):

A Is best treated with mannitol if the blood–brain barrier is impaired.
B May occur after suxamethonium.
C Can result in hypertension and bradycardia.
D Impairs cerebral perfusion pressure only after mean arterial pressure is reduced.
E Of more than 60 mmHg is irreversible.

230 The following are recommended in the management of a severe diffuse head injury:

A ICP between 20 and 40 mmHg.
B PaO_2 > 13 kPa.
C $PaCO_2$ between 3.0 and 4.0 kPa.
D Cerebral perfusion pressure > 100 mmHg.
E Jugular venous oxyhaemoglobin saturation > 85%.

231 In a neonate (full term):

A Systolic blood pressure is about 60 mmHg.
B The ductus arteriosus remains patent for up to 2 weeks after birth.
C Arterial hypoxaemia can reopen the ductus arteriosus.
D Compensatory mechanisms for hypotension are less efficient.
E A higher value of PaO_2 in the dorsalis pedis artery as compared to the right radial artery indicates persistent fetal circulation.

232 With regard to modes of ventilation in the management of anaesthesia for removal of a foreign body from the right main bronchus of a child aged 5 years:

A Rigid bronchoscopes are not equipped with the facilities to provide IPPV.
B IPPV could cause distal migration of the foreign body.
C Spontaneous ventilation can cause hyperinflation and pneumothorax if the foreign body produces a ball-valve action.
D IPPV is difficult due to narrow bronchoscopes and leaks around them.
E Muscle relaxation and IPPV are desirable as they produce excellent operative conditions.

229 A **False**   Mannitol should not be given if the blood–brain
                    barrier is suspected to be impaired as its leakage
                    and subsequent sequestration of fluid into the
                    interstitial space can actually increase ICP.
     B **True**
     C **True**   This is the characteristic haemodynamic change.
     D **False**   Cerebral perfusion pressure (CPP) = MAP – ICP
                    (if ICP > venous pressure).
     E **False**   Transient increases over this level are normal in
                    everyday activity.

230 A **False**   ICP should be maintained at a level < 25 mmHg.
     B **True**
     C **False**   Only moderate hyperventilation is recommended.
                    Therefore, $PaCO_2$ should be above 4 kPa.
     D **False**   Cerebral perfusion pressure of about 70 mmHg is
                    recommended.
     E **False**   The normal value for the jugular venous
                    oxyhaemoglobin saturation is 55–75% and it should
                    be maintained at this level.

231 A **True**
     B **False**   Functional closure occurs 10–15 h after birth and
                    anatomic closure occurs in 4–6 weeks.
     C **True**   As well as other conditions associated with
                    increased pulmonary vascular resistance.
     D **True**
     E **False** PaO_2 is higher in preductal arteries in persistent fetal
                    circulation.

232 A **False**   Jet injectors are often available.
     B **True**
     C **False**   This is a problem with IPPV.
     D **True**
     E **False**   Spontaneous ventilation is desirable.

233 **In a patient with a history of prior myocardial infarction:**

A Elective abdominal operation should be postponed for at least 6 months.

B Duration of thoracic surgery influences the risk of reinfarction.

C Intensive haemodynamic monitoring reduces the risk of reinfarction after non-cardiac surgery.

D Risk of reinfarction is the same whether it is single or triple vessel disease.

E Risk of reinfarction is not related to intraoperative hypertension or tachycardia.

234 **Intraoperative transoesophageal echocardiography is useful in monitoring for:**

A Left ventricular function.

B Valvular function.

C Air embolism.

D Intracardiac shunts.

E Haemodynamic parameters like cardiac output and ejection fraction.

235 **The following will decrease the outflow obstruction associated with hypertrophic cardiomyopathy:**

A Tachycardia.

B Hypovolaemia.

C β-blockade.

D CA^{2+} channel blockers.

E IPPV.

236 **A patient with a temporary transvenous pacemaker suddenly loses consciousness. ECG shows continuous pacing spikes but without capture. The heart rate is 40 beats.min^{-1}.**

A A likely cause is the displacement of the pacemaker electrode from the myocardium.

B Atropine or isoprenaline can be given in an attempt to increase the heart rate as an immediate, short-term measure.

C The stimulating electrode should be advanced until there is capture.

D Cardioversion should be attempted if other measures fail.

E An external pacemaker is of no use in this situation.

233   A **True**   Risk of reinfarction is over 20% in the first 3 months.
      B **True**   Upper abdominal or thoracic surgery of >3 h
                     duration increases the risk.
      C **True**
      D **False**   Triple vessel disease carries more risk.
      E **False**   Both increase risk.

234   A **True**
      B **True**
      C **True**
      D **True**
      E **True**

235   A **False**   Reduced diastolic time compromises diastolic filling
                     and this favours outflow obstruction.
      B **False**
      C **True**   Mild reduction of contractility relieves obstruction.
      D **True**
      E **False**   This has no effect alone.

236   A **True**
      B **True**   These may not be effective, though.
      C **True**
      D **False**   Cardioversion is not indicated, as this will not
                     increase the rate.
      E **False**   An external pacer should be used if other measures
                     fail to improve the heart rate.

237 **The following would help in diagnosing ventricular premature beats on ECG:**

A Premature positioning of the beat.
B Absent P wave.
C Normal QRS complex.
D Compensatory pause after the beat.
E ST segment in a direction opposite to the QRS complex.

238 **Anaesthesia and surgery may have adverse effects on renal blood flow due to:**

A Increased sympathetic activity.
B Increased secretion of antidiuretic hormone.
C Hypoxaemia.
D Pain.
E Increased plasma renin activity.

239 **Prior to liver transplant:**

A Renal function should be optimised.
B Liver enzymes should be corrected to normal.
C Nitrogen balance should be controlled.
D Ascites should be controlled.
E Infusion of blood products is contraindicated.

240 **In the regulation of bronchomotor tone:**

A β_1 receptors play a predominant role.
B Cyclic AMP acts as a second messenger.
C Parasympathetic influence antagonises sympathetic influence.
D Corticosteroids are effective owing to their anticholinergic effect.
E Antihistamines have no direct effect.

237 A **True**
     B **True**
     C **False**   Wide complexes.
     D **True**
     E **True**

238 A **True**
     B **True**
     C **True**   Increased sympathetic activity.
     D **True**   Increased sympathetic activity.
     E **True**   Consequence of the stress response.

239 A **True**
     B **False**   This is not achievable.
     C **True**
     D **True**
     E **False**   Coagulopathies may need to be treated using these
                       products.

240 A **False** β_2 receptors have a dilatory effect.
     B **True**   cAMP is a second messenger in β receptors.
     C **True**
     D **False**   Steroids reduce inflammation and sensitise
                       β receptors to β agonists.
     E **False**   Antihistamines reverse histamine-induced spasm.

Paper 7

241 The following conditions necessitate the preoperative placement of a cardiac pacemaker:

A Sick sinus syndrome.
B Acquired complete heart block.
C Marked sinus arrhythmia.
D First-degree heart block with left axis deviation.
E Asymptomatic bifascicular block.

242 Perioperative myocardial infarction:

A Is most common in the intraoperative period.
B Is best avoided by maintaining the heart rate and blood pressure at normal values for the population.
C Is no more likely after long operations than short operations.
D Is fatal in approximately 50% of cases.
E Is less likely in the presence of anaemia, reducing blood viscosity.

243 Regarding phaeochromocytoma:

A Orthostatic hypotension is common.
B β-blockade should be followed by α-blockade in preparation for surgery.
C Noradrenaline infusion is often required postoperatively.
D Hyperglycaemia is often seen postoperatively.
E Several weeks of preoperative normotension are required for normalisation of circulating blood volume.

244 Concerning lithium:

A It has a high therapeutic index.
B Common symptoms of toxicity include muscle weakness and facial flushing.
C It prolongs the action of suxamethonium.
D Preoperative i.v. fluids help to avoid lithium toxicity.
E Acute toxicity is treated with i.v. saline solution and osmotic diuresis.

Answers

241 A **True**
     B **True**   Congenital, complete heart block may not
                      necessitate placement of a pacemaker.
     C **False**   This is common in children and athletic young
                      adults.
     D **False**   Progression to serious conduction defect is rare.
     E **False**   Progression is rare. Symptoms of syncope,
                      palpitations or light-headedness necessitate a
                      pacemaker.

242 A **False**   It is most common in the postoperative period.
     B **False**   It is better to maintain these at normal values for the
                      patient.
     C **False**   It is more common after long operations, and after
                      abdominal or thoracic surgery.
     D **True**
     E **False**   Anaemia increases myocardial demand, while
                      reducing oxygen delivery.

243 A **True**   Due to the reduced circulating volume.
     B **False**   β-blockade should follow α-blockade because of the
                      risk of sudden heart failure.
     C **True**   Removal of the catecholamine-secreting tumour
                      may cause prolonged vasodilatation.
     D **False**   Hypoglycaemia is often seen.
     E **True**

244 A **False**   Lithium toxicity occurs at concentrations of
                      approximately 1.5 mmol.l^{-1}, while therapeutic
                      concentrations are 0.5–1.2 mmol.l^{-1}.
     B **False**
     C **True**   Probably through presynaptic inhibition of
                      transmitter synthesis and release.
     D **True**   Dehydration may dangerously increase plasma
                      levels.
     E **True**   Haemodialysis may be required in severe cases.

245 Regarding central venous pressure measurement:

A Trends in values are of little value in patients with valvular defects.
B The v wave represents atrial filling.
C Cannon v waves are seen in complete heart block.
D In the spontaneously breathing patient, CVP should be measured in mid-inspiration or mid-expiration.
E CVP measurement may facilitate microshock.

246 Regarding electroencephalography:

A Beta waveforms are characterised by high-frequency, low-amplitude activity.
B The cerebral function analysing monitor uses Fourier transformation to present data more meaningfully.
C EEG correlates well with imminent arousal.
D Seizure activity is seen on EEG with increasing doses of several inhalational anaesthetic agents.
E Spectral edge frequency is the EEG frequency below which 95% of activity is present.

247 Regarding the pharmacokinetic constants of i.v. induction agents:

A Thiopentone has α and β half-lives of approximately 2–7 and 42–59 min respectively.
B The systemic clearance of propofol is approximately 10 times greater than that of thiopentone.
C The α half-lives of propofol, methohexitone and ketamine are similar.
D 5β-pregnanolone has a similar systemic clearance to propofol.
E The α half-life of midazolam is approximately 10 times greater than that of propofol.

248 Regarding allergic reaction to i.v. induction:

A Allergic reaction to thiopentone is an IgE-mediated reaction with an incidence of approximately 1 : 10 000–1 : 15 000.
B Allergic reaction can occur without complement involvement.
C Allergic reaction to etomidate is very rare compared to other induction agents.
D Midazolam produces occasional complement-related allergic reactions.
E Change of formulation of propofol from Cremophor to Intralipid has reduced allergic reactions.

245 A **False**   Absolute values may be suspect, but trends are very useful.
     B **True**   It represents atrial filling against a closed tricuspid valve.
     C **False**   Cannon a waves are seen.
     D **False**   CVP should be measured at the end of expiration when intrathoracic and intrapleural pressures are zero.
     E **True**

246 A **True**   Typically, 14–30 Hz and <20 μV.
     B **False**   The compressed spectral array uses Fourier transformation.
     C **False**   Spectral edge frequency correlates weakly, but the other types of EEG do not.
     D **False**   This is only seen with one currently used agent, enflurane.
     E **True**

247 A **True**
     B **True**
     C **True**
     D **True**
     E **False**   It is 5–15 min, as compared to propofol's 1–4 min.

248 A **True**
     B **True**   Although this is rare.
     C **True**   The rate is between 1 : 50 000 and 1 : 450 000.
     D **False**   There have been no reported allergic reactions to midazolam.
     E **True**   Cremophor has been implicated in producing allergic reactions in combination with several drugs.

249 Concerning body temperature during anaesthesia:

A The thalamus controls body temperature by coordinating signals from many parts of the body.

B The thermoregulatory threshold is depressed in relation to the depth of anaesthesia.

C During normal surgical anaesthesia, the thermoregulatory threshold is reduced to approximately 34.5°C.

D During surgical anaesthesia in an operating room at 16°C, body temperature falls by 2–3°C in the first hour.

E The reduction in minimum alveolar concentration (MAC) during hypothermia is linearly related to the lipid solubility of the agent.

250 Regarding gastrectomy:

A It was more common in 1999 than 10 years previously.

B It is a high-risk procedure.

C It is a contraindication to epidural blockade.

D It may be performed as an emergency procedure.

E Patients always have an increased risk of aspiration pneumonitis.

251 Regarding cardiac risk assessment before vascular surgery:

A During dipyridamole–thallium scintigraphy (DTS), an area of delayed imaging indicates a previous infarct.

B It is dangerous and inappropriate to increase heart rate during DTS.

C Left ventricular function may be assessed using M-mode echocardiography.

D Left ventricular angioscintigraphy provides objective assessment of systolic function.

E The risks involved in measuring left ventricular ejection fraction make it a little-used preoperative evaluation.

252 Hypermagnesaemia:

A Is caused by renal failure.

B May be precipitated by the excessive use of diuretics.

C Causes prolongation of the P–R interval on the electrocardiogram.

D Causes tetany and muscle weakness.

E Has no effects on the CNS.

249 A **False** The hypothalamus is the area responsible for body temperature control.

B **True**

C **True**

D **False** Body temperature typically falls by 0.7–1.5°C in the first hour.

E **True** MAC of halothane thus falls 5% per 1°C for halothane and 2% per 1°C for cyclopropane.

250 A **False** Recognition of the aetiological role of *Helicobacter pylori* and the advent of H_2-blockers has made medical management more popular.

B **True** Patients may be bleeding, when mortality is 20%, or may have cancer and be in a poor physical state.

C **False** This may be a very useful means of postoperative analgesia.

D **True** Bleeding peptic ulcer may require emergency surgery. Adequate resuscitation is vital, even if a small delay in surgery is necessary.

E **False** Some may have an increased risk (e.g. bleeding peptic ulcer), but many have a normal cardiac sphincter and normal gastric contents.

251 A **False** This indicates an area of poor perfusion/ischaemia.

B **False** It improves sensitivity and may be accomplished by exercise or by upward tilting.

C **False** Two-dimensional echocardiography is more appropriate.

D **True**

E **False** It may be measured using two-dimensional echocardiography and is a useful predictor of perioperative morbidity and mortality.

252 A **True**

B **False** Diuretics typically cause hypomagnesaemia.

C **True** QRS prolongation and peaked T waves are also seen.

D **False** Muscle weakness is often seen but tetany is a feature of hypomagnesaemia.

E **False** Coma may ensue.

253 Non-pressurised ascent from sea level to 10 000 m above sea level causes:

A Immediate hyperventilation.
B A gradual increase in respiratory minute volume over the first few days at altitude.
C Acidification of the urine.
D A shift of the oxyhaemoglobin dissociation curve to the left.
E Clubbing of the fingers.

254 Portal hypertension:

A Results in oesophageal varices.
B Is caused by cystic fibrosis.
C May require liver transplant.
D Often results in abdominal ascites.
E Responds to systemic antihypertensive therapy.

255 Normal nutritional requirements include:

A 1 g.kg^{-1} nitrogen per day.
B At least 1000 kJ.kg^{-1} per day.
C 2 g.kg^{-1} lipid per day.
D 5 mmol.kg^{-1} sodium ions per day.
E $30-40 \text{ g.kg}^{-1}$ water per day.

256 $PaCO_2$:

A May be halved by doubling the minute volume.
B Is increased by a metabolic acidosis.
C Is reduced by increasing VO_2.
D Is reduced in uncomplicated carbon monoxide poisoning.
E Is calculated rather than measured directly by modern blood gas analysis machines.

257 During a stellate ganglion block, 3 ml of 0.5% bupivacaine are injected. The patient becomes drowsy and demonstrates slurred speech. Potential causes include:

A Syncopal episode.
B Vertebral artery injection.
C Subarachnoid anaesthesia.
D Epidural injection.
E Recurrent laryngeal nerve anaesthesia.

253 A **True** Hypoxaemia is the cause.
    B **True** As the kidneys correct the respiratory alkalosis, the stimulatory effect of hypoxaemia is potentiated.
    C **False** The kidneys excrete bicarbonate in an attempt to compensate for the respiratory alkalosis, alkalinising the urine.
    D **True** Hypocarbia is the cause. There is later a shift to the right as 2,3-DPG content of red cells is increased.
    E **True** Although this is rare and is associated with deterioration and severe mountain sickness.

254 A **True** Increased portal venous pressure distends the plexus running around the base of the oesophagus.
    B **True** Varices may also be seen.
    C **True** Although this is only useful if severe organ damage is isolated to the liver.
    D **True**
    E **False** Systemic antihypertensive agents do not cause portal venous dilatation.

255 A **False** Requirements are 1–2 g protein.kg^{-1} per day or 7–20 g nitrogen per day.
    B **False** 100 kJ.kg^{-1} per day.
    C **True**
    D **False**
    E **True**

256 A **True** Roughly: new $PaCO_2$ = current $PaCO_2$ × current minute volume/new minute volume.
    B **False** The two are independent.
    C **False** Increasing VO_2 with a constant respiratory quotient causes $PaCO_2$ to rise.
    D **False** This has no effect. The hypoxaemia caused by carbon monoxide poisoning does not usually cause hyperventilation.
    E **False** It is measured using the carbon dioxide electrode.

257 A **True** These symptoms may be associated with fainting.
    B **True** CNS toxicity is quite possible even with this small amount of local anaesthetic when injected directly into the arterial supply.
    C **True** The subarachnoid space is reachable with a 5 cm block needle during a stellate ganglion block.
    D **False** Although it is possible to inject into the epidural space during this block, epidural injection without i.v. or subarachnoid injection will not produce these symptoms.
    E **False** The patient would not become drowsy as a result of laryngeal nerve blockade.

258   Regarding a witnessed cardiac arrest:

A If ECG monitoring is not attached, a precordial thump is inappropriate.

B Adrenaline should be given once every 2 min until the blood pressure is over 50 mmHg systolic.

C Cardiac massage generates venous pressures almost as high as arterial pressures.

D If VF is diagnosed, defibrillations are given in sets of three without interruption.

E One should aim to maintain a normal PaO_2.

259   The volume of distribution of a drug:

A Determines its β half-life.

B May exceed total body water volume.

C Is larger for lipid-soluble drugs than for water-soluble drugs.

D Is calculated as: dose given/plasma concentration.

E Represents one or several body compartments.

260   Gastric contents:

A Whose pH is above 4 are unlikely to cause problems if aspirated into the lungs.

B Are consistently increased in volume even by minor trauma.

C Typically have a pH of less than 1.

D Are unlikely to be significant if the patient is hungry.

E Are more likely to be regurgitated following induction of anaesthesia by the obstetric patient than the non-pregnant patient.

261   Sweating during general anaesthesia may indicate:

A Hypocarbia.

B Hypoxia.

C Deep anaesthesia.

D Hypercapnia.

E Pain.

258 A **False**   In a witnessed arrest, when diagnosis is uncertain, a precordial thump should be used.
     B **False**   Once a pulse has been re-established, adrenaline should only be given as indicated.
     C **True**
     D **True**
     E **False**   100% oxygen should be given.

259 A **True** $t_{1/2\beta}$ = volume of distribution/clearance.
     B **True**   The volume of distribution is the volume that the drug would be dissolved in if it existed throughout the body at the concentration found in plasma. Fat-soluble drugs thus may have a volume of distribution larger than body volume.
     C **True**   See B.
     D **True**
     E **False**   It does not represent any body compartments. See B.

260 A **False**   A pneumonitis is still likely and severe hypoxaemia may occur if solids are aspirated.
     B **False**   Research suggests that gastric emptying continues though at a slower rate. Minor trauma may not affect emptying at all.
     C **False**   The pH is usually between 1 and 4.
     D **False**   There is no evidence that this is the case. Hunger has a complex aetiology that includes psychological factors.
     E **True**   Increased intra-abdominal pressure and impairment of the gastric cardiac sphincter make regurgitation more likely.

261 A **False**
     B **False**
     C **False**
     D **True**
     E **True**
Sweating during general anaesthesia is usually due to marked carbon dioxide retention, sympathetic stimulation or light anaesthesia.

262 Relaxation of the gravid uterus can be obtained by administration of:

A Halothane.
B Alfentanil.
C Ether.
D Spinal anaesthesia at a level of D10.
E Nitrous oxide and atracurium.

263 With regard to the myotomes of the lower limbs:

A L2/L3 extend the hip.
B L4/L5 flex the hip.
C L4/L5 dorsiflex the ankle.
D L3/L4 extend the knee.
E L5/S1 flex the knee.

264 The following are the sensitive tests to evaluate sympathetic block:

A Skin conductance response.
B Laser Doppler flowmetry.
C Sweat test.
D Change in skin colour.
E Change in skin temperature.

265 With regard to anxiolytic premedication in patients undergoing day-case surgery:

A A combination of pethidine and promethazine provides ideal conditions.
B Benzodiazepines and opiates delay gastric emptying.
C Oral midazolam can be used in children.
D Temazepam has the same half-life as lorazepam in children.
E Oral transmucosal fentanyl is superior to all other premedication drugs in children over 5 years of age.

266 With regard to the peripheral nociceptors:

A C fibres are associated with well-localised pain.
B Afferent stimuli from A-mechano-heat receptors travel in A fibres.
C C-polymodal receptors are non-myelinated C fibres.
D Inflammatory mediators sensitise these receptors, resulting in primary hyperalgesia.
E These receptors do not exhibit plasticity.

262 A **True**
     B **False**
     C **True**
     D **False**
     E **False**
General anaesthesia (including administration of volatile agents) will be necessary to provide uterine relaxation if the uterus remains firmly contracted around the placenta.

263 A **False**
     B **False**
     C **True**
     D **True**
     E **True**
In the lower extremity, flexion at the hip is achieved by L2 & L3 and extension by L4 & L5. At the knee L3 & L4 extend and L5 & S1 flex. At the ankle, dorsiflexion is achieved by L4 & L5 and plantar flexion by S1 & S2.

264 A **True**
     B **True**
     C **True**
     D **False**
     E **False**
Change in skin colour and temperature are quite subjective measures of sympathetic block and are therefore not as sensitive as the other three methods, which tend to be objective.

265 A **False**   Long duration of action; excessive sedation.
     B **False**   Benzodiazepines do not delay gastric emptying.
     C **True**
     D **False**   It is shorter.
     E **False**   Pruritus, nausea and respiratory depression are common side effects.

266 A **False**   These are associated with dull burning and poorly localised pain.
     B **True**
     C **True**
     D **True**
     E **False**   Plasticity (i.e. varying frequency of discharge to a constant stimulus) is an inherent property of nociceptive neurones.

267 Neonates:

A Are more resistant to opioids than older children.

B Require a lower concentration of local anaesthetic drug to block nerve conduction than do older children.

C Are not suitable for epidural or spinal anaesthesia.

D Are at greater risk of toxicity from local anaesthetics than older children.

E Have the same half-life for fentanyl as for morphine.

268 Appropriate strategies to manage a patient in septic shock include the following:

A Avoid invasive monitoring as far as possible.

B Filling pressures should be kept low to prevent ARDS.

C Blood culture and removal of the source of infection.

D Low SVR is best left untreated to reduce myocardial afterload.

E Antibiotic therapy should be withheld until culture reports are available.

269 With normocapnia ICP is increased after the administration of:

A Fentanyl.

B Lignocaine.

C N_2O.

D Isoflurane.

E Halothane.

270 Postoperative complications of carotid endarterectomy include:

A Labile blood pressure.

B Myocardial infarction.

C Stroke.

D Weakness of the tongue.

E Persistent hoarseness.

271 Neonates and infants are prone to develop hypothermia because:

A They have a large body surface area.

B The insulating subcutaneous fat layer is thin.

C Shivering is of little significance in heat production.

D Increasing the ambient temperature of the operating room is ineffective.

E Anaesthetics depress brown fat thermogenesis.

267 A **False**   They are more sensitive.
     B **True**
     C **False**   Spinal anaesthesia is quite commonly performed.
     D **True**
     E **False**   The half-life of fentanyl is less than that of morphine.

268 A **False**   Invasive monitoring allows early optimisation of
                    oxygen delivery.
     B **False**   Filling pressures need to be optimised for adequate
                    oxygen delivery.
     C **True**
     D **False**   Organ perfusion can be significantly improved by
                    treating a low SVR.
     E **False**   Antibiotics should be started empirically.

269 A **False**
     B **False**
     C **True**
     D **True**
     E **True**
     Only the inhalational agents are known to cause marked
     increases in ICP. Narcotics have minimal effect and lignocaine
     may actually reduce it.

270 A **True**   Carotid sinus mechanisms.
     B **True**   Labile haemodynamic conditions may contribute.
     C **True**
     D **True**   Caused by nerve damage.
     E **True**   Trauma to the laryngeal nerve supply is the culprit.

271 A **True**
     B **True**
     C **True**   Thermogenic shivering is not fully developed in
                    neonates.
     D **False**   The main mechanism of heat loss is by radiation and
                    increasing ambient temperature to thermoneutral
                    temperature helps to reduce the heat loss.
     E **True**

272 **In a patient with a large diaphragmatic hernia at birth:**
   A The degree of lung hypoplasia determines the outcome.
   B Fetal pattern of circulation may persist.
   C Tolazoline may be given to treat pulmonary hypertension.
   D Preoperative ventilation is not recommended as it may cause pneumothorax.
   E Passage of a nasogastric tube increases respiratory distress.

273 **The following preoperative factors contribute to increased mortality after CABG surgery:**
   A Reoperation.
   B Age of more than 50 years.
   C Females over 40 years of age.
   D Angina.
   E Concomitant mitral valve replacement.

274 **In the pericardial space:**
   A About 50–70 ml of fluid is normally present.
   B During spontaneous ventilation pressure increases during inspiration and decreases during expiration.
   C 250 ml of fluid will cause loss of cardiac silhouette in a chest radiograph.
   D Sudden accumulation of 150 ml of fluid can cause cardiac tamponade.
   E Accumulation of excessive fluid is reliably detected by echocardiography.

275 **In a hypertensive crisis:**
   A Diagnosis can only be made if diastolic blood pressure is above 160 mmHg.
   B Blood pressure should be rapidly normalised to prevent end-organ damage.
   C Cerebral autoregulation prevents any increase in cerebral blood flow.
   D Nitroprusside infusion is an effective form of treatment.
   E Intra-arterial pressure monitoring is not indicated.

272 A **True**
 B **True** This is due to increased pulmonary artery pressure.
 C **True**
 D **False** Children with large hernias usually require mechanical ventilation and stabilisation of the condition before surgery is contemplated.
 E **False** A gastric tube is indicated to relieve the distress.

273 A **True**
 B **False** Age of more than 70 years is associated with increased mortality.
 C **True**
 D **False** Most patients going for this surgery would have angina. Unstable angina, however, is a strong risk factor for mortality.
 E **True**

274 A **False** The normal figure is 20–25 ml.
 B **False** The converse is true; pressure stays subatmospheric throughout.
 C **True**
 D **True**
 E **True**

275 A **False** The arbitrary limit is 130 mmHg.
 B **False** The aim is prompt but gradual reduction of diastolic BP to 100–110 mmHg over a period of several minutes to several hours. A rapid decrease in BP can cause end-organ ischaemia.
 C **False** Cerebral blood flow autoregulation limits are usually crossed in a hypertensive crisis.
 D **True**
 E **False** Intra-arterial pressure monitoring is indicated, especially when vasodilators are used to control the BP.

276 **The following measures should be taken to prevent pacemaker malfunction due to electrocautery:**

A The ground plate should be placed away from the pulse generator.
B A unipolar form of electrocautery should be used instead of bipolar.
C Long, widely placed bursts are less risky.
D The electrocautery current should be kept to the minimum possible.
E A magnet should be placed on the pulse generator prophylactically.

277 **The side effects of amiodarone include:**

A Pulmonary fibrosis.
B Bradycardia.
C Gingival hyperplasia.
D Thyroid dysfunction.
E Corneal deposits.

278 **In a patient with chronic renal failure:**

A Cardiac output is decreased.
B Blood viscosity is decreased.
C Plasma proteins are elevated.
D Hyperventilation reduces oxygen delivery to tissues.
E Elevation in serum sodium precedes the elevation in H^+ ions.

279 **In a patient awaiting heart transplant:**

A Loop diuretics will reduce the preload.
B Digitalis is contraindicated.
C ACE inhibitors are useful in reducing the afterload.
D Mechanical circulatory support is contraindicated.
E Dobutamine and amrinone can provide inotropic support.

280 **The following cause a decrease in the diffusing capacity of the lungs:**

A Pulmonary oedema.
B Emphysema.
C Asthma.
D Anaemia.
E Lung collapse.

276 A **True**
     B **False**   A bipolar electrocautery is preferable.
     C **False**   Short bursts, 10 s apart, are recommended.
     D **True**
     E **False**   It should be kept handy in case the pacemaker starts malfunctioning.

277 A **True**
     B **True**
     C **False**
     D **True**
     E **True**

278 A **False**   Anaemia causes an increase in cardiac output.
     B **True**   Anaemia.
     C **False**   These are usually reduced.
     D **False**   The hyperventilation is an attempt to compensate for the metabolic acidosis.
     E **False** K^+ and H^+ ions are elevated earlier than Na^+.

279 A **True**
     B **False**   Digitalis may be indicated to optimise the mechanical efficiency of the failing heart.
     C **True**
     D **False**   This may be the only way to keep the patient alive.
     E **True**

280 A **True**   By increasing the alveolar–arterial distance.
     B **True**   Structural damage impairs diffusion.
     C **False**   Airway disease does not (in isolation) affect diffusion.
     D **True**   Because of reduced capacity to carry carbon monoxide.
     E **True**   By reducing the available lung surface.

Paper 8

281 Regarding patients with thyroid disease:

A Hypothyroidism increases the risk of awareness during general anaesthesia.
B Heart failure may be caused by hypo- or hyperthyroidism.
C Goitre may cause insurmountable respiratory obstruction following induction of anaesthesia.
D Thyroid storm may necessitate the administration of β-blockers and thyroxine.
E Expiratory retardation on flow-volume loops indicates tracheal compression by goitre.

282 Regarding aortic stenosis:

A The gradient across the aortic valve should be measured using cardiac catheterisation.
B An enlarged heart shadow is usually seen on the chest X-ray.
C A gradient of 20 mmHg across the valve indicates severe disease.
D Regional anaesthesia usually produces better cardiovascular conditions.
E Heart rate should be kept as low as possible intraoperatively to aid ventricular filling.

283 The obese patient:

A Is at greater risk to health from abdominal obesity than gluteal–femoral obesity.
B Suffers arterial desaturation more quickly than the non-obese patient.
C Has peripheral airway obstruction.
D Demonstrates longer duration of action of anaesthetic induction agents.
E Always has a smaller functional residual capacity than a non-obese patient of the same weight.

Answers

281 A **False** Anaesthetic requirements are reduced by hypothyroidism.
   B **True**
   C **True** This must be excluded before anaesthesia is commenced.
   D **False** Thyroid storm is not treated with thyroxine.
   E **False** Inspiratory retardation is more commonly a sign of extrathoracic tracheal compression.

282 A **False** Doppler cardiography is a much safer way to measure the gradient.
   B **False** Although the left ventricle is hypertrophied, a visibly enlarged heart is not visible until late in the disease.
   C **False** A gradient of 70–100 mmHg indicates a severe disease.
   D **False** Regional anaesthesia may produce cardiac decompensation if pronounced vasodilatation occurs.
   E **False** Heart rate is best maintained at normal values.

283 A **True** Free fatty acids are more easily mobilised from abdominal fat.
   B **True** The oxygen reserves in the FRC are reduced, and oxygen consumption is higher.
   C **True** Obese men show a 20% reduction in forced expiratory flow rates.
   D **False** Termination of action is generally unaffected.
   E **False**

284   Concerning benzodiazepines:

A They are muscle relaxants.
B They potentiate the effect of γ-hydroxybutyric acid by acting upon its receptor.
C Diazepam has, in common with midazolam, an active metabolite, desmethyldiazepam.
D Withdrawal of chronic benzodiazepine therapy causes convulsions.
E Overdose usually produces dangerous respiratory and cardiovascular depression.

285   Regarding the pulmonary artery catheter:

A It allows measurement of left ventricular filling pressure.
B It is necessary to allow estimation of pulmonary shunt fraction.
C It allows measurement of pulmonary physiological deadspace fraction without expired gas collection.
D It should be sited in West zone II.
E Monitoring for small rises in pulmonary artery occlusion pressure allows sensitive detection of myocardial ischaemia.

286   Concerning evoked potentials:

A Anaesthetic agents produce a decrease in latency of evoked potentials.
B Ischaemia produces the same effect as anaesthesia.
C Brain stem auditory evoked potentials are sensitive to anaesthesia and show a drop in amplitude with increasing depth of anaesthesia.
D Somatosensory evoked potentials give information about the posterior columns but little about the anterior cord.
E Middle-latency evoked potentials are more sensitive to anaesthesia than long- and short-latency responses.

287   The following factors reliably speed the induction of anaesthesia using a volatile agent:

A Hyperventilation.
B Increasing water solubility of the volatile agent.
C Hypovolaemia.
D Hypervolaemia with cardiac failure.
E The application of 10 cmH$_2$O positive end-expiratory pressure.

284 A **True**   Their effect is centrally mediated.
    B **True**
    C **False**   Desmethyldiazepam, while an active metabolite of
                 diazepam and other benzodiazepines, is not a
                 metabolite of midazolam.
    D **True**   Convulsions may result from benzodiazepine
                 withdrawal.
    E **False**   They are relatively safe in overdose.

285 A **False**   It allows indirect estimation of left ventricular filling
                 pressure.
    B **False**
    C **True**   Physiological deadspace fraction = 1 − (Barometric
                 pressure × CO_2 production)/(arterial CO_2 tension ×
                 Expired minute volume).
    D **False**   Ideally it should be sited in West zone III.
    E **False**   Myocardial ischaemia does produce rises in PAOP
                 due to changing ventricular compliance, but the
                 sensitivity of this method is inadequate to justify the
                 risk involved.

286 A **False**   They increase latency.
    B **True**   Ideally, anaesthetic agents should be constant
                 during monitoring of spinal cord function.
    C **False**   They are fairly resistant to anaesthesia.
    D **True**
    E **False**   Long-latency are the most sensitive, but are virtually
                 completely suppressed during anaesthesia.

287 A **True**
    B **False**   Equilibration of the alveoli is slowed by absorption
                 of agent into the blood.
    C **True**   Low cardiac output increases the rate of rise of
                 alveolar, and thus brain, tension.
    D **True**   See above.
    E **False**   In some patients this may increase minute volume,
                 but in most it will reduce it. The increase of the mean
                 pressure in the lungs has a minimal effect on
                 anaesthetic effect.

288   Concerning porphyria:

A Alcohol may precipitate porphyric crises.
B Acute attacks of porphyria cutanea tarda are not precipitated by drugs.
C Barbiturates and fentanyl constitute an acceptable anaesthetic for the porphyric patient.
D The non-depolarising muscle relaxants have been experimentally shown to be triggers of porphyria.
E All forms of porphyria result in elevated urinary 5-aminolaevulinic acid.

289   Concerning metabolic requirements during anaesthesia:

A During a 6 h preoperative period with no oral intake, a 70 kg patient will develop a water deficit of 630 ml.
B During prolonged anaesthesia, basal metabolic rate is typically reduced by 50%.
C Tissue oxygen delivery is maximised by replacing a blood loss of 30% circulating volume in the non-anaemic patient with crystalloids.
D Extracellular, non-intravascular fluid volume is reduced by surgery.
E A fall in core temperature of 3°C reduces metabolic water requirement by 20%.

290   Regarding pancreatic surgery:

A Pancreatitis causes hypercalcaemia.
B Vitamin K is occasionally required preoperatively even in the non-warfarinised patient.
C Carcinoma of the pancreas causes obstructive jaundice.
D Pancreatitis may cause a pancreatic cyst, requiring emergency drainage.
E Whipple's procedure is a pancreatico-duodenotomy.

291   A 45-year-old male has the following arterial blood gas results: PaO_2 7.8 kPa, $PaCO_2$ 7.6 kPa and pH 7.38.

A He has an acidosis.
B He has type II respiratory failure.
C Ventilatory failure secondary to myasthenia is a possible diagnosis.
D His base excess is less than 2.5 mmol.l^{-1}.
E Arterial oxygen saturation is approximately 90%.

288 A **True**   This is a common trigger.
     B **True**
     C **False** Barbiturates are potent triggers.
     D **False**
     E **False** Porphyria cutanea tarda does not result in elevated
                   urinary ALA levels.

289 A **True**   Water requirement for a resting adult is typically
                   1.5 ml.kg^{-1}.h^{-1}.
     B **True**   Hypothermia, the direct effect of anaesthetics and
                   artificial ventilation account for this.
     C **True**   The 'optimal' haematocrit is approximately 25–30%
                   when the reduction in blood viscosity increases
                   tissue oxygen delivery.
     D **True**
     E **True**   Values of 6–8 % per 1°C are quoted.

290 A **False** Hypocalcaemia may be caused by lipid soap
                   formation.
     B **True**   Biliary obstruction may derange hepatic synthesis of
                   clotting factors.
     C **True**   By obstructing the common bile duct.
     D **True**   Especially if the cyst is infected.
     E **False** It is a pancreatico-duodenectomy.

291 A **True**   He has a respiratory acidosis.
     B **False**
     C **True**   He has metabolic compensation, so the cause is
                   probably long-standing.
     D **False** This would be a normal base excess. He certainly
                   has a large base excess to compensate for this
                   respiratory acidosis.
     E **True**

292 In a 70 kg male during starvation:

A Glycogen stores last for approximately 1 week.
B Negative nitrogen balance is 5–35 g per day.
C Loss of 30% body weight only marginally affects chances of survival during illness.
D Liberation of energy from protein and fat is approximately 2000 kJ per day.
E Loss of 15% body weight may cause respiratory failure in a previously healthy individual.

293 Regarding the pulmonary artery:

A Vascular resistance decreases as cardiac output increases.
B Flow is less than in the aorta.
C Vascular resistance is approximately five times less than systemic vascular resistance.
D Vascular resistance is not affected by the application of positive end-expiratory pressure during mechanical ventilation.
E It has a lower mean intraluminal pressure than the right ventricle.

294 A 65-year-old man presents with COPD and a history of increasing SOB over 2 days. Arterial blood gas analysis is given: F_IO_2 0.4, PaO_2 6.5 kPa, $PaCO_2$ 8.5 kPa, pH 7.38, BE +6.0 mmol.l^{-1}.

A He has respiratory and ventilatory failure.
B He has respiratory mechanical failure.
C His hypercapnia is chronic.
D He has an alkalosis.
E His pulmonary shunt is >5%.

295 In a patient with acute tubular necrosis secondary to ongoing hypovolaemia:

A High-output renal failure is likely.
B If urinary urea concentration is <20 times plasma concentration then renal function is poor.
C Urinary sodium concentration is likely to be >20 mmol.l^{-1}.
D Haemofiltration should be instituted as soon as possible.
E The patient is likely to demonstrate a respiratory alkalosis.

292 A **False**   They are depleted after 1–2 days.
     B **True**
     C **False**   Survival is unlikely after this degree of weight loss during starvation.
     D **False**   It is approximately 7000 kJ per day.
     E **True**   Patients with this degree of weight loss due to starvation require feeding before weaning will be successful.

293 A **True**   This occurs because of recruitment of additional vessels and vascular distension.
     B **True**   Some aortic flow is diverted into vessels supplying the bronchi and ventricular muscle, emptying into the left ventricle.
     C **False**   SVR = 80 × (MAP − RAP)/CO ≈ 1360, while PVR = 80 × (MPAP − LAP)/CO ≈ 160.
     D **False**   PVR is increased by PEEP.
     E **False**   The mean pressure is higher. The pulmonary valve prevents backward flow.

294 A **True**   He has increased shunt and an inadequate ventilatory minute volume.
     B **True**   This means that he cannot manage to ventilate an adequate minute volume.
     C **True**   It probably is chronic. The metabolic compensation is the clue here.
     D **True**   He has a metabolic alkalosis.
     E **True**   A shunt of 5% is not large. This patient's shunt is approximately 50%.

295 A **False**   Urine output will decrease or even cease.
     B **True**   This is a useful objective measure in hypovolaemic patients.
     C **True**   Urine sodium concentration during hypovolaemia should normally be less than 20 mmol.l^{-1} because of the effects of aldosterone.
     D **False**   The hypovolaemia should be corrected and good renal perfusion restored. Haemofiltration may be required at a later stage if renal function does not recover.
     E **True**   Compensating for the metabolic acidosis due to the kidneys' failure to excrete protons.

296 Following emergency laparotomy for perforated large bowel, the following data are obtained: BP 80/55, CI 2.0 l.min⁻¹.m⁻², SVRI 1800 dyn.s.cm⁻⁵, CVP 0 mmHg, PCWP 2 mmHg.

A Septic shock is likely to be present.
B The first line of treatment should be i.v. adrenaline administration.
C Fluids should be rapidly infused.
D A noradrenaline infusion should be commenced.
E The patient is very unlikely to survive.

297 Concerning thoracic epidural anaesthesia:

A It carries less risk than lumbar epidural anaesthesia.
B It usually produces more hypotension than lumbar epidural anaesthesia.
C It is most difficult between T3 and T7.
D Dural puncture is less likely to result in spinal cord damage than in the lumbar region.
E Horner's syndrome may be seen with high epidural anaesthesia.

298 The following are preferred in the fluid resuscitation of the victim of major burns:

A Dextrose saline solution.
B Whole blood.
C Hypertonic saline.
D Plasma protein fraction.
E 10% dextrose solution.

296   A **True**   Although currently the patient is hypovolaemic.
      B **False**   This would be dangerous. Fluids are urgently
                      required.
      C **True**
      D **False**   If prolonged and used in the absence of fluid
                      resuscitation, this treatment may result in organ
                      failure and death.
      E **False**   There are no data to suggest this currently.

297   A **False**   The thoracic epidural space is thinner than the
                      lumbar space and the spinal cord may be damaged
                      inadvertently when performing thoracic epidural
                      anaesthesia.
      B **True**   Lumbar epidural anaesthesia tends to produce less
                      sympathetic blockade than thoracic because the
                      sympathetic outflow stops at approximately L2 in
                      the adult.
      C **True**   This is because of the steepness of inclination of the
                      spinous processes and the size of the intervertebral
                      foramina.
      D **False**   The spinal cord extends to approximately L2 in the
                      adult.
      E **True**   Blocking the sympathetic supply to one side of the
                      face causes Horner's syndrome. High thoracic
                      epidural anaesthesia, blocking the first few thoracic
                      roots, will cause this.

298   A **False**   Dextrose-containing solutions rapidly redistribute to
                      extravascular tissues, causing oedema and
                      intravascular hypovolaemia.
      B **True**   This causes minimal oedema and has an excellent
                      intravascular half-life, although it is not frequently
                      required acutely. There are obvious problems with
                      its use, including infection and cost.
      C **True**   This has been used successfully, reducing oedema
                      and thus improving tissue oxygen delivery.
      D **True**   This maintains intravascular oncotic pressure.
      E **False**

299 Regarding non-steroidal anti-inflammatory drugs (NSAIDs):

A They reduce prostaglandin synthesis.
B They increase substrate utilisation via the lipoxygenase pathway.
C They may cause renal damage via efferent arteriolar constriction.
D All NSAIDs have been implicated in causing Reye's syndrome.
E They most commonly cause bronchospasm via type IV hypersensitivity.

300 Surgical cross-clamping of the abdominal aorta:

A Will cause a sustained increase in cerebral blood flow.
B Is a useful manoeuvre in managing major haemorrhage from the splenic artery.
C May precipitate renal failure.
D Usually increases myocardial perfusion.
E May cause sudden death.

301 Gastric emptying time is increased by a standard dose of:

A Morphine.
B Methadone.
C Scopolamine.
D Thiopentone.
E Suxamethonium.

302 Lithium may cause:

A Sedation.
B Prolongation of the action of depolarising muscle relaxants.
C Prolongation of the action of non-depolarising muscle relaxants.
D Increased excretion of sodium.
E Reduced requirement of anaesthetics.

299 A **True**   They block the enzyme cyclooxygenase.
    B **True**   The arachidonic acid metabolites unused in the
                  synthesis are available for use in the alternative
                  lipoxygenase pathway.
    C **False**   They reduce the levels of protective prostacyclin in
                  the afferent arterioles of the kidneys.
    D **False**   Only aspirin has been implicated.
    E **False**   Asthmatic patients (especially those with nasal
                  polyps and atopic symptoms) may react with
                  bronchospasm to aspirin and other NSAIDs, but it is
                  rare. It occurs because of substrate diversion via the
                  lipoxygenase pathway, and only extremely rarely via
                  a type I (anaphylactic) hypersensitivity mechanism.

300 A **False**   Arterial pressure will fall quickly as cardiac output
                  and vascular resistance fall, and cerebral vascular
                  resistance will rapidly increase.
    B **True**   This may be life-saving, allowing time to isolate the
                  bleeding vessel.
    C **True**   Renal failure following open repair of ruptured
                  abdominal aortic aneurysms is often caused by
                  prolonged aortic cross-clamping.
    D **True**   The increase in diastolic pressure increases
                  perfusion. Unfortunately, myocardial oxygen
                  demand also increases markedly, and ischaemia is
                  often worsened unless arterial pressure is
                  dangerously low before cross-clamping.
    E **True**   Lethal pulmonary oedema may develop or the aorta
                  may tear causing fatal haemorrhage, especially if it
                  is atherosclerotic.

301 A **True**
    B **True**
    C **True**
    D **False**
    E **False**
Narcotics and antimuscarinic drugs significantly delay gastric
emptying time through different mechanisms of action.

302 A **True**
    B **True**
    C **True**
    D **False**
    E **True**
The association of sedation with lithium therapy suggests that
anaesthetic requirements for injected and inhaled drugs could
be reduced. Responses to depolarising and non-depolarising
neuromuscular blocking drugs may be prolonged in the
presence of lithium.

303 The following can be used safely for i.v. regional anaesthesia:

A 1% bupivacaine.
B 0.25% bupivacaine.
C 0.5% prilocaine.
D 0.5% lignocaine.
E 2% lignocaine.

304 With regard to local anaesthetic activity:

A Lipid solubility correlates with potency.
B pK_a is relevant to solubility and onset of action.
C pH of tissues determines the degree of ionisation.
D Action is better in acidotic tissues.
E Lignocaine has quicker onset than bupivacaine.

305 When compared with endotracheal intubation, insertion of the laryngeal mask is associated with:

A Easier isolation of the airway.
B Less pressor response.
C Same degree of increase in intraocular pressure.
D Requirement for similar depth of anaesthesia.
E Increased risk of regurgitation of gastric contents.

306 The phenomenon of secondary hyperalgesia:

A Refers to altered perception of peripheral stimuli due to widening of the receptive field.
B Can result from repeated C fibre afferent input.
C Refers to lowered threshold of pain in the area of tissue damage.
D Is probably modulated by NMDA receptor.
E Has nothing to do with the second messenger system in the dorsal horn.

303 A **False**
     B **False**
     C **True**
     D **True**
     E **False**
Approximately 40 ml local anaesthetic is required. Bupivacaine is contraindicated because of lower threshold of heart to produce arrhythmias with bupivacaine. Arrhythmias caused by bupivacaine are refractory to the treatment.

304 A **True**
     B **True**
     C **True**
     D **False**
     E **True**
Local anaesthetics are weak bases and therefore ionise in the acidic media, leaving a smaller proportion of the non-ionised, active form for the blocking action.

305 A **False**   The airway is not isolated with LM.
     B **True**
     C **False**   Rise in intraocular pressure is less with LM.
     D **False**   A lighter level of anaesthesia is needed for LM.
     E **True**

306 A **True**   The phenomenon is that of central sensitisation.
     B **True**
     C **False**   This results from primary hyperalgesia.
     D **True**
     E **False**

307 Regarding myalgia after suxamethonium:

A A patient who is ambulatory within 24 h is more likely to suffer.

B The severity of pain correlates with the severity of post-suxamethonium fasciculations.

C Pretreatment with a non-depolarising neuromuscular blocker reduces the incidence of fasciculations but not that of myalgia.

D Pretreatment with diclofenac is effective in reducing the incidence.

E Pretreatment with calcium gluconate is a reliable preventive measure.

308 Management of a restless patient in the recovery room may include:

A Relieving gastric distension.

B Correction of hypoxia.

C Relieving bladder distension.

D Relieving pain.

E Treatment with a short-acting benzodiazepine.

309 In the management of increased ICP:

A Hyperventilation is effective within 5 min.

B Osmotic diuretics work quicker than the loop diuretics.

C Steroids are effective within 30 min.

D Ketamine is recommended if all measures are ineffective.

E Plateau waves appear after successful treatment.

310 During carotid endarterectomy:

A Hypotension is required to prevent rupture of the carotid artery at the time of application of the clamp.

B Reflex bradycardia as well as tachycardia may be seen.

C Stump pressure of >50 mmHg is a reliable predictor of adequate CBF.

D Carbon dioxide should be moderately increased to allow better perfusion of the brain.

E EEG is a sensitive method to detect cerebral ischaemia.

311 Regarding water and electrolyte handling in children:

A Two-thirds of total body water is extracellular at birth.

B GFR is highest at birth and then decreases gradually to the adult value by 2 years of age.

C Capacity to preserve sodium is less.

D Drugs eliminated by the kidneys are more easily excreted at a younger age.

E Neonates have a reduced capacity to reabsorb bicarbonates.

307 A **True**
    B **False**   There is no firm correlation.
    C **False**   Both fasciculations as well as myalgia are
                     attenuated.
    D **True**   But not ketorolac.
    E **False**   There is some effect, but it is unreliable.

308 A **True**
    B **True**
    C **True**
    D **True**
    E **False**   This usually increases restlessness, unless the
                     primary cause is treated.

309 A **True**
    B **True**   Osmotic diuretics are effective in 15 min and loop
                     diuretics take 30–45 min.
    C **False**   Steroids take hours before they are effective.
    D **False**   Ketamine increases ICP.
    E **False**   These indicate critically reduced intracranial
                     compliance.

310 A **False**   Blood pressure should be maintained at normal
                     level.
    B **True**
    C **False**   Recent evidence suggests that there is no correlation
                     between stump pressure and CBF.
    D **False**   Normocapnia should be maintained.
    E **False**   Transcranial Doppler ultrasonography and jugular
                     venous oxygen saturation may give some indication
                     but none of the tests is very specific.

311 A **True**
    B **False**   GFR is low at birth and this limits the ability of
                     young children to handle fluid overload.
    C **True**   This is because of smaller length of the loop of
                     Henle.
    D **False**   Excretion depends on GFR.
    E **True**   This is due to diminished activity of carbonic
                     anhydrase in the distal tubule.

312 Recommended perioperative management of a child with a large gastroschisis includes:

A Prevention of hypothermia.

B Prevention of septicaemia.

C Use of a muscle relaxant and IPPV using nitrous oxide and an inhalational agent as part of a balanced anaesthetic technique.

D Optimising the condition of the patient even if surgery is marginally delayed.

E Planning a prolonged postoperative stay in the ICU.

313 Increased morbidity risk after cardiac surgery is seen in patients with:

A New-onset angina.

B Increasing severity of angina.

C Silent ischaemia on preoperative ECG examination.

D Diffuse disease of coronary vasculature.

E More than 50% decrease in the left main coronary artery diameter.

314 Pathophysiological changes in cardiac tamponade include:

A Increased central venous pressure.

B Normal right atrial pressure.

C Normal left atrial pressure.

D Increased pulmonary artery occlusion pressure.

E Increased systemic vascular resistance.

315 The following complications can be expected after treatment with ACE inhibitors:

A Hypokalaemia.

B Rebound hypertension.

C Proteinuria.

D Angioedema.

E Congestive heart failure.

316 With regard to anaesthetic management of a patient with a cardiac pacemaker:

A Suxamethonium and etomidate should be used with extra caution.

B A preoperative chest X-ray is recommended.

C A magnet should be available with programmable pacemakers.

D Postoperative shivering has extra hazards.

E Atropine and isoprenaline should be available.

312 A **True**
     B **True**
     C **False**   Nitrous oxide should be avoided to prevent
                     intestinal distension.
     D **True**
     E **True**

313 A **True**
     B **True**
     C **True**
     D **True**
     E **True**
     All these factors increase the incidence of perioperative
     myocardial infarction.

314 A **True**
     B **False**   Right atrial pressure is increased. A persistent and
                    progressive increase in pericardial pressure leads to
                    equalisation at about 20 mmHg of right and left
                    atrial pressures and pulmonary artery end-diastolic
                    and occlusion pressures.
     C **False**
     D **True**
     E **True**   This is a secondary effect of reduced cardiac output.

315 A **False**   Hyperkalaemia is more likely, especially with renal
                    insufficiency and with concurrent use of potassium-
                    sparing diuretics.
     B **False**   This is not expected from use of drugs that act
                    independent of the autonomic nervous system.
     C **True**
     D **True**   This may cause upper airway obstruction.
     E **False**

316 A **True**   Muscle movements associated with shivering,
                    suxamethonium, etomidate-induced myoclonus and
                    seizures can inhibit some pacemakers and result in
                    their malfunction.
     B **True**   This may detect any break in the pacemaker electrode.
     C **False**   Magnets cause random reprogramming of some
                    pacemakers, which can be dangerous. Magnets
                    should only be used with non-programmable
                    pacemakers.
     D **True**
     E **True**

317   Causes for third-degree heart block include:

A Digoxin toxicity.
B Myocardial infarction.
C Ankylosing spondylitis.
D Cocaine overdose.
E Hyperkalaemia.

318   A pulmonary artery catheter in a patient with alcoholic cirrhosis is likely to show:

A Elevated filling pressure and low cardiac output (CO).
B Normal filling pressure, elevated CO and low systemic vascular resistance (SVR).
C Elevated filling pressure, normal CO and elevated SVR.
D Low filling pressure, elevated CO and elevated SVR.
E Normal filling pressure, normal CO and extremely elevated SVR.

319   The following features are characteristic of chronic renal failure:

A Hypertension.
B Hypochromic megaloblastic anaemia.
C Hypoparathyroidism with hypocalcaemia.
D Shift of the oxyhaemoglobin dissociation curve to the right.
E Increased plasma bicarbonate.

320   The ratio of peak expiratory to peak inspiratory flow is reduced in:

A Fixed upper airway obstruction.
B Extrathoracic upper airway obstruction.
C Intrathoracic upper airway obstruction.
D Lower airway obstruction.
E Obesity.

317 A **True**
     B **True**
     C **True**
     D **False**   Tachydysrhythmias are common.
     E **True**

318 A **False**   Possible at the advanced stage when
                     cardiomyopathy develops.
     B **True**   The usual picture is that of hyperdynamic
                     circulation.
     C **False**   SVR is unlikely to be elevated.
     D **False**
     E **False**

319 A **True**
     B **False**   Normocytic normochromic.
     C **False**   Hyperparathyroidism with hypercalcaemia is
                     characteristic.
     D **True**
     E **False**   Reduced bicarbonate (metabolic acidosis).

320 A **False**   There will be a decrease in both inspiratory and
                     expiratory flow rates of similar degree.
     B **False**   This will selectively decrease inspiratory flow.
     C **True**
     D **True**
     E **False**   Both inspiratory and expiratory flows will be
                     affected.

Paper 9

321 Malignant hyperthermia:

A Is carried on the short arm of chromosome 19.
B Is transferred in an autosomal dominant fashion, and expression is complete.
C Is more common in children than in adults.
D Is more common in the presence of osteogenesis imperfecta.
E May be triggered by competitive muscle relaxants.

322 Patients with mitral stenosis:

A Have almost always suffered rheumatic fever in the past.
B Demonstrate a reduced pulmonary compliance.
C Often have a loud second heart sound.
D Tolerate elevations in heart rate during anaesthesia poorly.
E Are best managed with positive pressure ventilation because of its beneficial effect on pulmonary vascular resistance.

323 Concerning human immunodeficiency virus (HIV):

A 80% of occupational exposure is via needlestick injury.
B Serum conversion after needlestick injury is 20–70 times more likely for hepatitis B than for HIV.
C HIV is a retrovirus, causing depletion of helper T lymphocytes.
D Kaposi's sarcoma may cause difficulty in airway management.
E Admission to the ITU may be necessary postoperatively.

324 Concerning glucocorticoids:

A They cause sodium and potassium retention.
B Patients taking steroids regularly require additional perioperative steroids because of their inability to absorb their usual oral dose.
C They often mask the signs of sepsis and peritonism.
D To mimic the normal response to major surgery, approximately 300 mg of hydrocortisone is required in the first 24 h following surgery.
E They may precipitate diabetes mellitus.

Answers

321   A **False**   It is carried on the long arm of chromosome 19.
      B **False**   Expression is incomplete.
      C **True**   In children, 1 : 15 000, while in adults, 1 : 50 000.
      D **True**   It is also more common with scoliosis, strabismus,
                      myotonia and dystrophies.
      E **False**   These may be safely used. Suxamethonium and
                      volatile agents are potent triggers.

322   A **True**   Although only 50% will give a history of it.
      B **True**   This is due to long-term effects on the lungs.
      C **True**   This is the pulmonary sound, made louder by
                      pulmonary hypertension.
      D **True**   Tachycardia reduces the already impaired ventricular
                      filling.
      E **False**   This may increase resistance, further impairing left
                      ventricular filling.

323   A **True**
      B **True**   Seroconversion for HIV is 0.5%, while for hepatitis B
                      it is 20–35%.
      C **True**
      D **True**   The larynx is involved in 20% of patients with
                      Kaposi's sarcoma.
      E **True**   Malnutrition is common, as is immunosuppression.
                      These patients may have a life expectancy of several
                      years.

324   A **False**   They weakly stimulate potassium excretion through
                      their mineralocorticoid effect.
      B **False**   The requirement for additional steroids is not
                      because of an inability to absorb the usual dose.
      C **True**
      D **False**   The dose required to mimic the normal response is
                      approximately 100–200 mg.
      E **True**

325 Regarding insertion of a pulmonary artery catheter (PAC):

A Pulmonary infarction may be precipitated.
B Insertion of a PAC reduces mortality in the critically ill.
C Ventricular stroke work is calculated from the arterial pressure, pulmonary artery occlusion pressure (PAOP) and stroke volume.
D Cardiac index and systemic vascular resistance index are calculated as the cardiac output and SVR divided by the body surface area.
E A left atrial catheter allows more accurate measurement of cardiac output than a pulmonary artery catheter.

326 Concerning the measurement of cerebral blood flow:

A Xenon washout is an accurate and established method.
B Transcranial Doppler gives an accurate value for cerebral blood flow velocity.
C The middle cerebral artery is easy to locate for use with transcranial Doppler.
D Distal carotid stump pressure provides information about the adequacy of collateral flow during carotid endarterectomy.
E Near infrared spectroscopy penetrates the skull and provides information about regional cerebral oxygenation.

327 Thiopentone:

A Is an oxybarbiturate.
B Influences the function of the GABA receptor.
C Is in common use as a 5% solution.
D Has a pH of 12.5 in its commercially available form.
E Is stored in nitrogen to prevent oxidation.

328 Concerning inhalational anaesthesia:

A The time constant for nitrous oxide uptake into the vessel-rich group is considerably shorter than in the fat compartment.
B The vessel-rich group (comprising 9% of body weight) receives 75% of the cardiac output.
C The equilibration time constant for desflurane is the same for the fat group and the muscle group.
D Of all the body compartments, fat takes the longest to equilibrate for all the volatile agents.
E Over-pressure is particularly important for agents with a low blood:gas partition coefficient.

325 A **True**   This is a recognised complication.
     B **False** There is no consistent evidence of this.
     C **True**   LVSW = (MAP – PAOP) × SV × 0.0136 g.m^{-1}.
     D **False** CI = CO/BSA; SVRI = SVR × BSA.
     E **False** A left atrial line does not allow cardiac output measurement.

326 A **True**
     B **True**   But it cannot measure total flow.
     C **True**   It is located at the temple.
     D **True**   Although there are frequent false positives and false negatives.
     E **True**

327 A **False** Methohexitone is an oxybarbiturate. Thiopentone is a thiobarbiturate (containing sulphur).
     B **True**   This may be the basis of its action.
     C **False** It is most commonly used as a 2.5% solution.
     D **False** It has a pH of 11.
     E **False** It is stored in nitrogen to prevent formation of the free acid by reaction with atmospheric carbon dioxide.

328 A **True**   It is quoted as 1.3 min as compared to 100 min.
     B **True**   It comprises brain, heart, kidneys, liver, gut and endocrine glands.
     C **False** Fat: 1350 min; muscle: 49 min.
     D **True**   This is due to the high solubility and the low blood flow.
     E **False** It is important for the soluble agents.

329 The following are found in patients with inflammatory bowel disease:

A Abnormal pulmonary function tests in 50% of patients.
B Impaired absorption of drugs.
C Vocal cord oedema.
D Increased incidence of malignant hyperpyrexia.
E Clotting defects in 15% of patients.

330 During hepatic surgery:

A Hepatic metastases from bowel tumour are not an indication for hepatic surgery.
B Veno-venous bypass preserves renal function worse than cross-clamping the inferior vena cava.
C Atracurium is preferable to vecuronium.
D Disseminated intravascular coagulation is diagnosed by a reduction in platelet count.
E Clinically apparent hypocalcaemia often occurs.

331 A 74-year-old female has the following blood gas results: F_IO_2 0.8, PaO_2 40 kPa, $PaCO_2$ 5.2 kPa and HCO_3^- 16 mmol.l^{-1}.

A She has an inappropriate respiratory minute volume.
B Her pulmonary shunt fraction is over 50%.
C Persistent vomiting could explain these blood gas results.
D She is likely to be hypokalaemic.
E Serum proton concentration is less than 40 nmol.l^{-1}.

332 The following are part of a suitable daily feeding regime for a 70 kg patient:

A 7.5 g of protein.
B 150 mmol sodium.
C 125–200 kJ.kg^{-1} per day.
D Intralipid 10%.
E 30–45 ml.kg^{-1} per day of water.

329 A **True**
     B **True**   Intestinal fibrosis may hinder absorption of orally
                    administered drugs.
     C **True**   This responds to steroids.
     D **False**   There is no evidence of this.
     E **False**   Clotting may be affected during very severe crises,
                    but not otherwise.

330 A **False**   Resection of isolated metastases increases median
                    survival times.
     B **False**   Veno-venous bypass permits free perfusion of the
                    renal bed.
     C **True**   It does not rely upon hepatic clearance for its
                    elimination.
     D **False**   Platelet count will fall in the absence of DIC.
                    Fibrinogen degradation products (FDPs) and
                    D-dimers should be measured.
     E **False**   Although minor fluctuations in serum calcium may
                    be seen secondary to citrate toxicity following
                    massive blood transfusion, it is rarely clinically
                    apparent.

331 A **True**   Her $PaCO_2$ is 5.3 kPa while her HCO_3^- is low,
                    implying a metabolic acidosis. She should be
                    hyperventilating to compensate.
     B **False**   She has an elevated shunt fraction, but nowhere
                    near 50%.
     C **False**   This would cause an alkalosis and would not usually
                    cause the elevation in shunt.
     D **False**   Metabolic acidosis often causes hyperkalaemia as
                    potassium ions and protons are exchanged at cell
                    surfaces and in the renal tubules.
     E **False**   The low HCO_3^- implies metabolic acidosis in the
                    presence of normal carbon dioxide tension. Her
                    proton concentration is thus elevated.

332 A **False**   70–140 g of protein are required.
     B **True**
     C **True**
     D **True**   This provides fats, cholesterol, energy and
                    phosphate.
     E **True**   More is required in the catabolic, burned, pyrexial or
                    septic patient.

333 Myocardial oxygenation is consistently increased by:

A An increase in respiratory minute volume.
B Systemic vasoconstriction.
C Blood transfusion.
D Administration of an increased inspired oxygen fraction.
E Aortic valvular regurgitation.

334 Hepatic cirrhosis:

A Results in irreversible damage to the liver.
B Is caused most commonly by hepatitis in the UK.
C May be managed with immunosuppressive agents.
D Is associated with hyponatraemia and hyperkalaemia.
E May be induced by anaesthetic agents.

335 With regard to intracranial pressure measurements following head injury:

A Extradural lines give the most accurate estimation of intracranial pressure.
B All intracranial pressure monitoring lines should be equipped with a flushing device.
C A rise in intracranial pressure to >30 mmHg during coughing is normal.
D Lundberg A waves are a normal finding.
E Intracranial pressure is reduced by total body cooling.

333 A **False**   This shifts the oxyhaemoglobin dissociation curve to the left, potentially reducing oxygen release to the myocardium, and may provoke a reduction in coronary vessel calibre and cardiac output. It may occasionally improve myocardial oxygenation by increasing PaO_2 when it is low (e.g. due to shunting or low inspired oxygen fraction).

B **True**   Afterload and oxygen demand may be increased, but diastolic pressure rises, increasing myocardial perfusion.

C **False**   This will usually improve myocardial oxygenation in the anaemic patient, but elevation of haemoglobin concentration above 100 g.l^{-1} will increase blood viscosity, potentially reducing myocardial oxygen delivery.

D **True**

E **False**   This increases LVEDP and thus reduces myocardial blood flow.

334 A **True**   By definition the damage is irreversible. Fibrous bands are laid down.

B **False**   It is most commonly caused by alcohol abuse in the UK.

C **True**   Those aetiologies of an autoimmune nature may respond.

D **False**   It causes secondary hyperaldosteronism, resulting in hypokalaemia.

E **True**   Halothane can cause hepatitis and subsequently cirrhosis.

335 A **False**   They are prone to blockage and damping. Intraventricular lines are the most accurate, but most dangerous.

B **False**   Flushing these lines may produce dangerous peaks in ICP if intracranial compliance is low.

C **True**   It may rise to over 60 mmHg during coughing or straining.

D **False**   They indicate elevated ICP and impaired compliance.

E **False**   Cooling may reduce cerebral metabolic rate and thus cerebral damage, but ICP is unaffected.

336 Halothane hepatitis:

A Occurs more commonly in children than in adults.
B Occurs in 1 in 5000 halothane anaesthetics.
C Is more common in the obese undergoing anaesthesia.
D Is related to the extent of trifluoroacetic acid production.
E May result in fatal hepatic failure due to cirrhosis.

337 Regarding the provision of anaesthesia via a circle breathing system:

A A closed system has no input or output.
B A closed system has no flow through the scavenging tubing.
C Soda lime is used more quickly with low flows than with high flows.
D Sevoflurane must not be used in circle systems because of substance A production.
E Low flows in a circle system result in maximal humidification of inspired gases.

338 Midazolam:

A Is a water-soluble benzodiazepine.
B Produces retrograde amnesia.
C Acts synergistically with fentanyl in induction of anaesthesia.
D Acts quickly because of its lipid solubility.
E May produce respiratory arrest.

339 Regarding the saturated vapour pressure (SVP) of water:

A It is 6.7 kPa at 37°C.
B It is affected by salts dissolved in it.
C It is the pressure at which water is in solid, liquid and gaseous forms simultaneously.
D It is unaffected by temperature.
E If breathing air at sea level, tracheal oxygen tension is approximately $(21 - SVP_{H_2O})$ kPa.

336 A **False**   The incidence in children is 1 : 200 000 and in adults 1 : 35 000.
    B **False**   See above.
    C **True**   This may be due to the increased likelihood of the accumulation of dangerous halothane metabolites.
    D **True**   It is thought that this metabolite causes the hepatitis.
    E **True**   Although this outcome is rare.

337 A **False**   Even a closed system requires input of oxygen at the rate of the patient's oxygen consumption (approximately 3 ml.kg^{-1}.min^{-1}).
    B **True**   All the delivered oxygen is consumed and all the produced carbon dioxide is absorbed.
    C **True**   High flows may flush some carbon dioxide from the system, thus preserving the soda lime.
    D **False**   There is no evidence of clinical problems in humans, and sevoflurane may be used.
    E **True**   Soda lime becomes hot during use, and the patient's exhaled water is preserved in the circuit.

338 A **True**   At physiological pH its structure changes, and the imidazole ring opens, rendering it water-, and thus blood-, soluble.
    B **False**   There is no evidence, other than anecdotal, that retrograde amnesia is produced by midazolam. Lorazepam may produce a small degree of retrograde amnesia.
    C **True**   The effect of a combination of the two is greater than the sum of their effects alone. Synergistic action is greater than additive action.
    D **True**   High lipid solubility allows rapid passage across the blood–brain barrier.
    E **True**   Although the benzodiazepines are relatively safe in overdose (compared to opioids), in very large overdoses they cause death by respiratory depression.

339 A **True**   This is the pressure exerted by vapour in equilibrium with its liquid phase. It is dependent on temperature and the purity of the liquid. It is independent of ambient pressure.
    B **True**   See A. The SVP of an impure liquid is lower than that of a pure liquid (e.g. salt water vs. pure water).
    C **False**   See A.
    D **False**   SVP rises as temperature rises until SVP equals atmospheric pressure, at which point the liquid boils. Water thus boils at a lower temperature at altitude, making a good cup of tea a rarity at the top of Everest.
    E **False** $P_{tracheal}O_2 = F_IO_2 \times (Pb - SVP_{H_2O}) = 21\% \times (101.3 - 6.7) = 19.86$ kPa.

340 The Severinghaus electrode:

A Measures proton concentration.
B Contains a bicarbonate solution.
C Has a quicker response time than the H^+ electrode.
D Is accurate to less than <1 Pa.
E Is no longer in common use.

341 The consequences of hyperventilation include:

A Cerebral ischaemia.
B Decreased mitochondrial NADH.
C Increased brain lactate production.
D Increased cerebral oxygen consumption.
E Reduced cerebral autoregulation.

342 Fat embolism is associated with:

A Appearance of fat globules in the urine.
B Confusion.
C Presence of fat in retinal vessels.
D Petechiae.
E Hypoxia.

343 The epidural space:

A Is between the dura mater and the subarachnoid mater.
B Contains spinal roots, blood vessels and fat.
C Extends from foramen magnum to L1.
D Has the ligamentum flavum as its posterior border.
E Is easier to locate in the thoracic region using the midline approach.

340 A **True**   Carbon dioxide reacts with water to form protons
              and bicarbonate. Electrodes surround pH-sensitive
              glass within a bicarbonate solution.

     B **True**   See A.

     C **False**   Carbon dioxide must diffuse through a semi-
              permeable membrane before it reacts with the
              bicarbonate solution and the proton concentration is
              then measured.

     D **False**   It is accurate to approximately 130 Pa, but this
              accuracy is not often seen clinically owing to micro-
              holes in the membrane or serum protein deposition.

     E **False**   It is still widely used in measuring carbon dioxide
              tension in blood.

341 A **True**
     B **False**
     C **True**
     D **False**
     E **False**

Hyperventilation for short periods is safe, provided there is no
significant cerebral vascular pathology. Hyperventilation with
$PaCO_2$ of less than 3 kPa can cause intense vasoconstriction
leading to compromised blood flow. This may cause an increase
in NADH and a decrease in oxygen consumption. Hypocarbia
can increase the width of autoregulatory plateau.

342 A **True**
     B **True**
     C **True**
     D **True**
     E **True**

The classic finding in fat embolism is the appearance of
petechial haemorrhages in the capillary plexus of the dermis.
Emboli may appear within the retinal vessels, and there may be
streaks of haemorrhage throughout the retina as well as macular
oedema.

343 A **False**
     B **True**
     C **False**
     D **True**
     E **False**

The epidural space is between the bony ligaments and the dura
mater and extends from the foramen magnum to sacral hiatus.
In the thoracic region, because of the angulation of the spinous
processes of the vertebrae, it is easier to locate this space
through the paramedian approach.

344 Pain carried by autonomic fibres is characterised by the following:

A Precise localisation.
B Sharp and definite in character.
C Representation at cortical levels.
D May be referred to other parts of the body.
E Easily treated with nerve block.

345 Propofol is the induction agent of choice in day-case anaesthesia because:

A It has a shorter elimination half-life than any of the currently available i.v. agents.
B It is associated with 'clear-headed' recovery.
C It has insignificant cardiovascular effects.
D It has insignificant respiratory effects with a dose of <3 mg/kg.
E It has a lesser incidence of excitatory phenomenon than thiopentone.

346 The following have an inhibitory influence on pain transmission in the dorsal horn:

A Substance P.
B Calcitonin.
C GABA.
D Endogenous serotonin.
E Acetylcholine.

347 The following have been implicated in the development of alveolar atelectasis after upper abdominal surgery:

A Increased inspired oxygen.
B Large tidal volumes.
C Absence of sighs.
D Treatment with narcotics.
E Diaphragmatic dysfunction.

348 The following factors can increase the risk of postoperative sepsis:

A Old age.
B Invasive monitoring.
C Cirrhosis.
D Steroids.
E Cytotoxic drugs.

344 A **False**
     B **False**
     C **False**
     D **True**
     E **False**
     Precise localisation, sharpness, cortical representation and lack of referral are typical of the pain carried by the somatic fibres. Autonomic pain reception is weak, poorly localised and primarily at the cord or reflex level.

345 A **True**
     B **True**
     C **False**   Induction causes a significant decrease in blood pressure that is mainly due to vasodilatation.
     D **False**   Suppression of laryngeal reflex and apnoea are well known.
     E **False**   Thiopentone is not associated with any excitatory phenomenon.

346 A **False**   Substance P and calcitonin have excitatory effects.
     B **False**
     C **True**
     D **True**
     E **True**   Other substances with inhibitory influence include α_2 agonists and endogenous opioids.

347 A **True**
     B **False**   Small tidal volumes are more likely to be a cause.
     C **True**   This is more common after narcotic treatment.
     D **True**
     E **True**   This takes at least 48 h to recover.

348 A **True**   Compromised immune system.
     B **True**
     C **True**   Compromised immunity.
     D **True**   These lower the immunity.
     E **True**

349 Cerebral blood flow autoregulation:

A Preserves cerebral perfusion pressure despite changes in MAP between 50 and 150 mmHg.

B Is impaired to a greater degree by i.v. rather than inhalational anaesthetics.

C Is only minimally affected by narcotics.

D Is preserved in hypertensive patients.

E Is mainly mediated by sympathetic fibres.

350 Regarding controlled hypotension with the use of vasodilators:

A It can cause an increase in CBF and ICP despite a reduction in BP.

B Mean arterial pressure of 45 mmHg less than the preoperative value is acceptable.

C Blood pressure in the circle of Willis is higher than that in the radial artery.

D Nitroprusside infusion should not exceed 1.5 mg.kg^{-1} in 1 h.

E It predisposes brain tissue to retractor anaemia.

351 For scheduled routine surgery:

A The recommended time for restriction on intake of clear fluids and milk is 2 h in a neonate.

B Solids should be restricted for 4 h in children up to 6 months of age.

C Runny nose due to an allergic disease is an absolute contraindication for general anaesthetic.

D Preferably 1 month should elapse after respiratory tract infection.

E Haemoglobin of 120 g.l^{-1} is normal at 3 months of age.

352 Tracheo-oesophageal fistula:

A Is usually diagnosed a few days after birth once problems with breathing develop.

B May require preoperative gastrostomy if gastric distension is life-threatening.

C Has less than 60% chance of survival with the commonest variety in a full-term neonate without associated abnormalities and pulmonary complications.

D Has its commonest site of communication in the proximal part of the trachea.

E Most commonly has an H type communication between oesophagus and trachea.

349 A **True**
    B **False**   Inhalational anaesthetics are potent in impairing cerebral autoregulation.
    C **True**
    D **True**   Although it may be effective at a higher range of arterial pressure.
    E **False**   Response is initially myogenic and later metabolic.

350 A **True**   Due to cerebral vasodilatation.
    B **False**   MAP should be maintained within 25% of preoperative value.
    C **False**   It is possible only in the Trendelenburg position.
    D **True**   To prevent build-up of cyanide.
    E **True**

351 A **False**   2 h for clear fluids and 4 h for milk.
    B **True**
    C **False**   It is not contraindicated in the absence of an exacerbation.
    D **True**
    E **True**

352 A **False**   It is usually diagnosed soon after birth owing to inability to pass a stomach tube or difficulty in feeding.
    B **True**
    C **False**   Chances of survival are almost 100%.
    D **False**   Fistula is usually at the carinal end of the trachea.
    E **False**   The commonest variety is a blind upper oesophageal pouch and a fistula connecting the stomach to the trachea.

353 Presence of the following would confirm impaired left ventricular function:

A Ejection fraction of <40%.
B PCWP > 18 mmHg.
C LVEDP > 18 mmHg.
D Left ventricular wall dyskinesia.
E Essential hypertension.

354 The following can lead to diagnosis of cardiac tamponade:

A Decreased voltage on ECG.
B Pulsus paradoxus.
C Kerley B lines on chest radiograph.
D Kussmaul's sign.
E Increased vascular markings in the upper lung zones on chest radiograph.

355 Orthostatic hypotension is a well-known complication with:

A Potassium-sparing diuretics.
B ACE inhibitors.
C Clonidine.
D Methyldopa.
E Prazosin.

356 Regarding protamine administration:

A 1 mg should be given for each 200 units of heparin.
B It can increase pulmonary artery pressure.
C Hypotension can occur.
D Anaphylaxis is possible in patients taking insulin preparations.
E Slow administration is recommended.

357 Recognised pulmonary changes in a patient with cirrhosis include:

A Arterial hypoxaemia and hyperventilation.
B Pleural effusion.
C Increased functional residual capacity.
D Depressed hypoxic pulmonary vasoconstriction.
E Platypnoea.

353   A **True**
      B **False**   Raised PCWP is not confirmatory as it may be seen
                       with mitral valve disease as well.
      C **True**
      D **True**
      E **False**   This may cause hypertrophy, but function remains
                       unaffected until a very advanced stage.

354   A **True**
      B **True**
      C **False**   Total lung water is not usually increased.
      D **True**   Venous pressure increases during inspiration.
      E **False**   Vascular markings are usually unchanged.

355   A **False**
      B **False**   These do not have primarily autonomic effects.
      C **True**   Due to autonomic effects.
      D **True**   See C.
      E **True**   See C.

356   A **False**   Recommended dose is 1 mg for every 100 units of
                       heparin.
      B **True**   By increasing pulmonary vascular resistance.
      C **True**   Due to peripheral vasodilatation.
      D **True**
      E **True**   See C.

357   A **True**   This is mainly due to marked A–V shunting of the
                       blood.
      B **True**
      C **False**   FRC may be reduced due to ascites.
      D **True**   Due to circulating inhibitors of HPV which are
                       normally metabolised by the liver.
      E **True**   Because of attenuated HPV, the patient can become
                       short of breath in the upright position (platypnoea)
                       owing to gravity-induced pooling of blood in the
                       bases of the lungs.

358 **Hepatic blood flow is significantly decreased by:**
   A Epidural anaesthesia.
   B Spinal anaesthesia.
   C Hypoxia.
   D Isoflurane.
   E Halothane.

359 **In the intraoperative management of a patient undergoing liver transplant:**
   A Invasive monitoring is not required routinely.
   B Moderate hypothermia (33–34°C) is desirable.
   C Acidosis should be allowed to correct itself.
   D Nitrous oxide increases the risk of air embolism.
   E Dopamine or mannitol is recommended to maintain adequate renal blood flow.

360 **The following will result from parasympathetic stimulation of the bronchi:**
   A Increased airway resistance.
   B Increased alveolar compliance.
   C Increased elastic work of breathing.
   D Increased secretions.
   E Increased resistive work of breathing.

358 A **True**
     B **True**
     C **True**
     D **True**
     E **True**

359 A **False**   This is mandatory.
     B **False**   Normothermia should be maintained.
     C **False**   Acidosis should be aggressively treated.
     D **True**
     E **True**   Hepatorenal shutdown is common.

360 A **True**
     B **False**   Autonomic influences have no direct effect on
                     alveolar compliance.
     C **False**   Elastic work of breathing is a function of compliance.
     D **True**
     E **True**   Due to increased airway resistance.

Paper 10

361 Regarding haemoglobinopathies:

A Sickle cell disease phenotype may be caused by a variety of genotypes.

B The HbS gene is present in approximately 30% of the UK and USA populations.

C The HbC gene is as common as the HbS gene.

D Anaemia, bony deformities and cardiac dysfunction are relatively common in sickle cell disease.

E Sickle cell disease may be encountered in patients of Greek, Indian, Afro-Caribbean and Italian descent.

362 Regarding cardiomyopathy:

A Functional regurgitant valves are common in the restrictive variety.

B It may present with massive hypertrophy on electrocardiography.

C It may be caused by parasitic infection.

D The hypertrophic form may be caused by Friedreich's ataxia.

E Patients with restrictive cardiomyopathy should receive positive pressure ventilation under general anaesthesia.

363 Concerning hyperparathyroidism:

A It results in osteoporosis.

B Peptic ulceration is common as a result of excessive gastrin production.

C Lengthening of the Q–T interval on electrocardiography is a sign of hypercalcaemia.

D Reduction of plasma calcium levels is accomplished with volume expansion and loop diuretics.

E Corticosteroids are of no value in acutely lowering plasma calcium levels.

Answers

361 A **False**   Sickle cell disease is caused by the HbSS genotype.
   B **False**   10%.
   C **False**   Its prevalence is about 2%.
   D **True**   Although there is considerable variation in clinical severity.
   E **True**   It may also be found in the southern USA.

362 A **False**   They are fairly common in the dilated variety.
   B **True**   Although even hypertrophic cardiomyopathy does not always show hypertrophy on ECG.
   C **True**   Trypanosomiasis may cause a cardiomyopathy.
   D **True**   These patients may develop severe left ventricular outflow obstruction.
   E **False**   This may cause immediate cardiac arrest due to vasodilatation and reduced venous return.

363 A **False**   Osteopenia is seen owing to increased bone resorption.
   B **True**
   C **False**   The Q–T interval may be shortened, although this is not common.
   D **True**
   E **False**   They may be useful, as may calcitonin.

364 Regarding oral hypoglycaemic agents:

A The sulphonylureas act by increasing peripheral sensitivity to insulin.
B Sulphonylureas have the advantage of being effective even in the presence of minimal β cell function.
C Biguanide hypoglycaemic agents inhibit hepatic gluconeogenesis.
D All oral hypoglycaemic agents inhibit the absorption of glucose from the gut.
E Metformin, being long-acting, may be given once daily.

365 Concerning cardiac output:

A It may be measured continuously using the Fick principle.
B When using the thermodilution method, the fluid should be as cold as possible.
C Accuracy and reproducibility are improved by averaging three thermodilution measurements.
D Recirculation of dye during dye-dilution cardiac output measurement is not a practical problem.
E Cardiac output = (mean arterial pressure − right atrial pressure) × 80 / systemic vascular resistance (dyn.s.cm^{-5}).

366 Regarding measurement of neuromuscular block:

A Supramaximal stimuli risk skin burns and nerve damage.
B Train-of-four stimulation should be repeated no more often than every 3 min.
C The train-of-four ratio is the ratio between T1 and the twitch height before blockade.
D The train-of-four uses four stimuli at 4 Hz.
E The post-tetanic count uses 1 Hz stimuli 3 s after a 5 s 50 Hz tetanus.

367 Methohexitone:

A Is more potent than thiopentone.
B Is a weaker acid than thiopentone.
C Is proconvulsant and is thus useful in providing anaesthesia for electroconvulsive therapy.
D Is methylated.
E Has four optical isomers.

364 A **False**   They act by increasing insulin secretion.
     B **False**   They require residual β cell function.
     C **True**   They also inhibit glucose absorption and increase
                     peripheral utilisation.
     D **False**   Only the biguanides do this.
     E **False**   It is usually given three times daily.

365 A **True**   Continuous arterial and mixed venous oximetry
                     allow continuous cardiac output measurement.
     B **False**   Ice-cold fluid can cause arrhythmia. Room
                     temperature is adequate.
     C **True**
     D **False**   Mathematical compensations have to be made for
                     this.
     E **True**

366 A **False**   They should be used in order to recruit all nerve
                     fibres.
     B **False**   A minimum period of 12 s is adequate to avoid local
                     reversal and neurotransmitter depletion.
     C **False**   It is the ratio between T1 and T4.
     D **False**   The train-of-four uses four stimuli at 2 Hz.
     E **True**

367 A **True**   Typical induction dose is 1.5 mg.kg^{-1} as compared to
                     3–6 mg.kg^{-1} for thiopentone.
     B **True**   Its pK_a is 7.9. This accounts for its greater potency.
     C **True**   Although the seizures it may provoke occur after
                     large doses.
     D **True**
     E **True**

368 Regarding the volatile anaesthetic agents:

A At a given partial pressure, the concentration of halothane in blood is greater than that of isoflurane.

B At a given partial pressure, brain concentration of halothane is lower than that of enflurane.

C The mixed venous partial pressure of volatile agents is always lower than the arterial partial pressure.

D Total body uptake of isoflurane during the first hour of anaesthesia with a constant inspired concentration is over twice that in the second hour.

E 5–10 ml.min^{-1} of nitrous oxide is lost through the skin of an adult when the alveolar concentration is 70%.

369 Bowel preparation preceding surgery:

A Frequently causes hyperkalaemia.

B Takes approximately 2 h.

C May cause surgery to be postponed.

D Consists of enemas only.

E Virtually guarantees an empty stomach.

370 Concerning splenectomy:

A It reduces the patient's resistance to non-encapsulated organisms.

B It is used in the treatment of thrombocytopenia.

C Patients undergoing elective splenectomy will often require perioperative steroid cover.

D Streptococcal vaccine is required after surgery.

E Platelet administration, if required, should always be given before the splenic artery is clamped.

371 A 52-year-old male presenting for bowel surgery has the following blood results: Na$^+$ 128 mmol.l^{-1}, K$^+$ 2.8 mmol.l^{-1}, Urea 14 mmol.l^{-1}, glucose 12 mmol.l^{-1}.

A Treatment with thiazide diuretics may have caused the abnormalities.

B If he is taking digoxin, it should be stopped immediately.

C His hyponatraemia should be treated before surgery.

D Secondary hyperaldosteronism could explain these results.

E He is dehydrated.

368 A **True**   Halothane has a higher blood:gas partition coefficient.
     B **False**   Halothane is more lipid-soluble than enflurane (as evidenced by its lower MAC value).
     C **False**   Once delivery of agent has halted washout from tissues occurs, causing mixed venous tension to rise above arterial tension.
     D **False**   Uptake differs remarkably little, of the order of 10–20%.
     E **True**

369 A **False**   There is loss of relatively potassium-rich fluid from the bowel.
     B **False**   Total preparation takes 1–2 days.
     C **True**   The patient's electrolytes may be severely deranged.
     D **False**   Oral medication is also required.
     E **False**   The gastric volume is unaffected. An empty stomach is almost never seen.

370 A **False**   It reduces the patient's resistance to encapsulated organisms such as *Pneumococcus* and *Haemophilus influenzae*.
     B **True**
     C **True**   These patients often have haematological problems and may have received high-dose or long-term steroids.
     D **False**   Pneumococcal vaccine is required.
     E **False**   They may be withheld until the artery is clamped to prevent platelet consumption by the spleen.

371 A **True**   Loop diuretics may produce a similar picture.
     B **False**   Although signs of toxicity should be sought, and his serum potassium should be treated as soon as possible.
     C **False**   His hyponatraemia is appropriate in response to his elevated urea and glucose levels. Plasma osmolality is normal.
     D **False**   Hyperaldosteronism causes hypokalaemia but does not cause any of the other observed abnormalities.
     E **False**   His osmolality is at the bottom of the normal range. His hyperuricaemia is caused by drugs or mild renal failure.

372 Concerning the administration of stored blood:

A Blood stored for 2 weeks has only half of its initial platelet count.
B Cryoprecipitate may be used to correct deficiencies of factor VII.
C Metabolism of citrate after blood transfusion commonly causes a metabolic alkalosis.
D Immediately following transfusion, arterial oxygen saturation is often higher even in the absence of a change in oxygen tension.
E Stored blood has a much higher potassium concentration than blood in vivo and this is exacerbated on rewarming.

373 Regarding blood types:

A No ABO antigens are expressed on cells in type O blood.
B Six genotypes determine the four phenotypes in the ABO blood group system.
C H antigen is expressed on all red cells.
D A and B antigens are peculiar to red cells.
E Rhesus antibodies occur naturally in most people.

374 Rheumatoid arthritis:

A Is inherited as an autosomal recessive.
B May affect any joint.
C Always causes a vasculitis.
D May affect the larynx.
E Is more commonly juvenile in onset.

375 The following cause difficulty in weaning a patient from mechanical ventilation:

A An elevated VO_2.
B Vital capacity 10–20 ml.kg^{-1}.
C Anaemia.
D Pulmonary deadspace of 10%.
E True cord oedema.

372 A **False**   There are virtually no functioning platelets.
    B **False**   Deficiencies of factor VIII are treated with
                  cryoprecipitate.
    C **True**   Although a metabolic acidosis is more commonly
                  seen during the acute phases of massive blood
                  transfusion.
    D **True**   The transfused red cells are low in 2,3-DPG and thus
                  bind oxygen avidly.
    E **False**   Rewarming blood causes cells to recommence
                  metabolic processes and potassium is transported
                  back into cells.

373 A **True**   Anti-A and anti-B antibodies are present in type O
                  serum, however.
    B **True**   Genotypes are AA, BB, AB, AO, BO, OO, while
                  phenotypes are A, B, AB, O.
    C **True**   A and B antigens are formed from substance H.
                  H antigen is expressed to a variable degree, but is
                  always present.
    D **False**   They may be found on white cells, platelets, and
                  epidermal and endothelial cells.
    E **False**   They may occur naturally, but are very rare.
                  Sensitisation is usually required (e.g. haemolytic
                  disease of the newborn is caused by rhesus D
                  sensitisation of the mother).

374 A **False**   It is HLA-DR4 linked.
    B **True**   It typically commences with tender, swollen hands
                  and then progresses to larger joints.
    C **True**   Although this may not be clinically apparent.
    D **True**   The arytenoids may be affected.
    E **False**   Peak onset is in the fourth decade.

375 A **True**   This places greater demands upon the respiratory
                  and cardiovascular system.
    B **False**   This is adequate to allow weaning, although once
                  extubated the patient may not cough adequately.
    C **True**   If moderate to severe, this places greater demands
                  upon the cardiovascular and respiratory systems.
    D **False**   This is a small value and would not impair weaning.
    E **False**   Weaning is unaffected. Extubation may be
                  dangerous.

376 Inhalational induction:

A Is hastened by the simultaneous administration of carbon dioxide.
B Requires venous access to be established first.
C Is hastened by a low cardiac output.
D With desflurane is faster than with sevoflurane.
E Is most usefully performed using a closed breathing system.

377 Regarding the provision of anaesthesia for emergency caesarean section:

A Spinal anaesthesia may not be used because it is slower than general anaesthesia.
B Any induction agent except ketamine may be used.
C The use of opioids at induction is associated with lower Apgar scores.
D A small dose of suxamethonium should be used so that its duration is short.
E The average blood loss during emergency caesarean section is 500 ml.

378 Regarding the following arterial blood gas results: PaO_2 5.5 kPa, $PaCO_2$ 6.1 kPa, pH 7.1, BE −7 mmol.l^{-1}:

A These are typical venous results.
B There is a respiratory alkalosis and a metabolic acidosis.
C HCO_3^- concentration is likely to be high.
D Pulmonary embolus is likely.
E These results are typical of a patient post-pneumonectomy.

376 A **True**   As long as the same concentration of volatile agent
                   is delivered, carbon dioxide will increase respiratory
                   minute volume and thus anaesthetic uptake.

    B **False**   This is ideal, providing the possibility of
                   administration of i.v. drugs if required, but
                   inhalational induction may be performed because
                   venous access cannot be obtained.

    C **True**   Paradoxically. Alveolar concentration builds up more
                   quickly, and, of the reduced cardiac output, a
                   fractionally greater amount goes to the brain.

    D **False**   Although the blood:gas partition coefficient of
                   desflurane (0.42) is lower than that of sevoflurane
                   (0.6), desflurane's irritant smell makes it a difficult
                   and slow agent to perform inhalational induction.

    E **False**

377 A **False**   Spinal anaesthesia is not necessarily slower than
                   general anaesthesia. In addition, the safety benefits
                   for mother and baby count for more than saving a
                   small amount of time.

    B **False**   The induction agent should be cardiostable and
                   short acting. The baby should not be excessively
                   sedated by it and it should have no adverse effects
                   upon uterine tone. Thiopentone is an appropriate
                   agent.

    C **True**   It is thus unwise to use opioids at induction. The
                   hypertensive response to intubation may be
                   obtunded in the pre-eclamptic patient with
                   magnesium or a small dose of short-acting opioid
                   (such as alfentanil).

    D **False**   An adequate dose should be used. Use of small
                   doses is associated with failure to intubate.

    E **False**   The average blood loss is over 1 litre, although
                   much of this is from the placental content.

378 A **False**   Venous base excess is typically greater than
                   -2.5 mmol.l^{-1}.

    B **False**   There are respiratory and metabolic acidoses.

    C **False**   It will be raised by the hypercapnia but will be
                   depressed to a greater degree by the metabolic
                   acidosis.

    D **False**   Hypercapnia is rare in pulmonary embolus, as is
                   metabolic acidosis. If PE precipitated these gases,
                   then the patient is in an extremely critical state.

    E **False**   These results are not typical.

379 The following are true of flow:

A Laminar flow rate is proportional to the third power of the radius.
B Turbulent flow is more likely in dense fluids.
C Laminar flow is favoured in vessels of large radius.
D Turbulent flow is more influenced by viscosity than is laminar flow.
E Turbulent flow is more likely in the trachea than in the bronchioles.

380 Constant output of volatile anaesthetic agent by modern vaporisers is maintained by:

A A water-filled heatsink.
B Bubbling the fresh gas flow through the volatile liquid.
C Baffles.
D Compensation for changes in ambient pressure.
E Automatic adjustment of the splitting ratio.

381 Regading methaemoglobinaemia:

A It is a complication of prilocaine local anaesthesia.
B It is treated with administration of methylene blue.
C 5–10% methaemoglobinaemia causes symptoms.
D It can be reconverted to haemoglobin by oxidising agents.
E It confounds pulse oximeter readings.

379 A **False**   Laminar flow rate = $\pi \times P \times r^4 / 8 \times \eta \times l$ (π is 3.141596, P is the pressure gradient, r is the radius, η is the viscosity, l is the length).

   B **True**   Reynolds' number = $v \times \rho \times r / \eta$ (v is the flow velocity, ρ is the density, r is the radius, η is the viscosity). In cylindrical tubes, if the value exceeds 2000, turbulent flow is likely.

   C **False**   See B.

   D **False**   Turbulent flow rate is proportional to the square root of the pressure gradient, the square of the radius and is inversely proportional to the density of the fluid.

   E **True**   See B. The radius of the trachea is larger.

380 A **False**   This method has been used in the past (e.g. Boyle's bottle and EMO), but metal heatsinks are more convenient and have been used more recently.

   B **False**   This was used previously (e.g. Boyle's bottle), but is no longer used.

   C **True**   This ensures maximal saturation of the fresh gas with volatile agent by encouraging turbulent flow.

   D **False**   There is no such compensation. At 2 atmospheres ambient pressure, the delivered partial pressure of the agent is unchanged, but the concentration is halved. Fortunately, the clinical effect of the volatile agent is related to its partial pressure, so vaporisers may be used at varying atmospheric pressures with some impunity.

   E **True**   The temperature of the volatile liquid (whose SVP is varying with temperature) determines the splitting ratio required to produce the required output. This is often accomplished using a bimetallic strip that bends due to the differing coefficients of thermal expansion of the two metals.

381 A **True**
   B **True**
   C **False**
   D **False**
   E **True**
Prilocaine, nitrites, sulphonamides and phenacetin can all cause methaemoglobinaemia. Levels of less than 20% rarely cause symptoms. It is reconverted to haemoglobin by reducing enzymes, ascorbic acid, glutathione or methylene blue.

382 The features of aspiration pneumonitis include:

A Tachypnoea.
B Persistent cyanosis.
C Distinctive ECG changes.
D Tachycardia.
E Wheeze.

383 For hypotension following subarachnoid block:

A A decrease in mean arterial pressure of 40% is acceptable.
B The immediate priority is to increase the contractility of the heart.
C α agonists are the vasoconstrictors of choice if hypotension is associated with tachycardia.
D Restoration of preload is sufficient in many cases.
E Use of crystalloids is contraindicated.

384 The triple airway manoeuvre includes:

A Lifting the chin.
B Head tilt.
C Forward displacement of the jaw.
D Opening the mouth.
E Airway suction.

385 With regard to the use of inhalational agents in children:

A Induction with halothane is smoother than that with isoflurane.
B Desflurane is more acceptable than halothane for induction.
C Sevoflurane has lower solubility in blood than desflurane.
D Cyclopropane is least soluble in blood when compared to isoflurane, desflurane or sevoflurane.
E Nitrous oxide is least soluble in blood when compared with any of the available agents.

386 With regard to the opioid receptors:

A β-endorphins are the endogenous agonists at μ receptors.
B μ and δ receptor agonists act by depolarising the nerve terminal.
C Agonists at μ receptors are effective by opening the K^+ channels.
D Kappa receptor agonists are effective by closing Ca^{2+} channels.
E Opioids may act to inhibit the inhibitory pathways, leading to excitatory phenomena.

382 A **True**
     B **True**
     C **False**   There are no distinctive ECG changes caused by
                     aspiration.
     D **True**
     E **True**

383 A **False**
     B **False**
     C **True**
     D **True**
     E **False**
     A decrease in mean arterial pressure of 20–25% is tolerated by
     most vital organs in healthy subjects. For hypotension following
     subarachnoid block the immediate priority is to increase the
     preload. This is sufficient in many cases. Both crystalloids and
     colloids can be used to correct the preload. In case vasopressors
     are considered, ephedrine is the drug of choice if hypotension is
     associated with bradycardia. However, in case the hypotension
     is associated with tachycardia, α-stimulators such as
     methoxamine are the vasoconstrictors of choice.

384 A **False**
     B **True**
     C **True**
     D **True**
     E **False**

385 A **True**
     B **False**   Like isoflurane, desflurane is an irritant to the upper
                     airway.
     C **False**
     D **False**   The blood:gas partition coefficient for desflurane is
                     0.42.
     E **False**   Desflurane is currently the least soluble in blood.

386 A **True**
     B **False**   Agonists at these receptors open K^+ channels. Efflux
                     of K^+ results in hyperpolarisation of the nerve
                     terminal, which becomes refractory to afferent
                     stimuli.
     C **True**
     D **True**
     E **True**   This explains nausea, vomiting and rarely
                     antinociception seen with opioids.

387 Recognised risk factors for development of pulmonary embolism after surgery are:

   A Malignancy.
   B Congestive heart failure.
   C Obesity.
   D Hip surgery.
   E Ageing.

388 Known complications of hypothermia in the postoperative period are:

   A Onset of new seizure activity.
   B Increased oxygen consumption.
   C Acute renal failure.
   D Bleeding diathesis.
   E Delayed recovery of consciousness.

389 The following are early reliable indicators of venous air embolism:

   A Mill-wheel murmur.
   B Precordial Doppler signal.
   C A sudden fall in end-tidal carbon dioxide.
   D Hypotension.
   E Cyanosis.

390 Concerning the Glasgow Coma Scale after head injury:

   A It provides a reproducible assessment of brain injury.
   B A score of 6 indicates severe injury.
   C The higher the score the more severe the injury.
   D An extensor motor response scores more than the flexor response.
   E Eye opening to speech scores more than spontaneous eye opening.

391 Neonates handle drugs differently from adults because of:

   A Lower hepatic clearance.
   B Lower renal clearance.
   C Higher protein binding.
   D Smaller proportion of body water.
   E Diminished enzyme activity.

387 A **True**
     B **True**
     C **True**
     D **True**
     E **True**

388 A **False**   Patients may remain unconscious.
     B **True**   This can increase by up to 500% during shivering.
     C **False**
     D **True**
     E **True**

389 A **False**   It is a late indicator of a massive air embolus.
     B **True**
     C **True**
     D **False**   A late indicator.
     E **False**   A late indicator.

390 A **True**
     B **True**   A score of 9 or less indicates severe injury.
     C **False**   The reverse is true.
     D **False**
     E **False**

391 A **True**
     B **True**
     C **False**   Albumin and α_1-acid glycoprotein have diminished
                     drug-binding capacity.
     D **False**   The proportion of body water is higher.
     E **True**

392 With regard to pyloric stenosis:

A It is seen more often in male infants at 2–5 weeks of age.
B Emergency surgery is warranted as soon as the diagnosis is made.
C The infant is depleted of hydrogen, chloride, potassium and sodium ions.
D The associated metabolic abnormality is hypokalaemic, hypochloraemic acidosis.
E Rapid sequence induction with cricoid pressure is one of the recommended techniques.

393 In a patient with significant aortic stenosis:

A Angina may be associated.
B LVEDP is likely to be increased.
C Coronary perfusion pressure is likely to be reduced.
D Both diastolic and systolic functions are likely to be affected.
E Coronary angiogram may be normal.

394 Failure of the left ventricular myocardium results in:

A A lower stroke volume at a given end-diastolic pressure.
B A rate-treppe phenomenon.
C Higher LVEDP and normal PCWP.
D Increased inotropic response to β agonists.
E Increased total lung water.

395 Side effects of β-blockers include:

A Congestive heart failure.
B Raynaud's phenomenon.
C Bronchospasm.
D Decreased systemic vascular resistance.
E Hyperglycaemia.

396 The following are features of aortic stenosis:

A Increased incidence of sudden death.
B Triad of angina, dyspnoea and syncope.
C Angina in the absence of coronary artery disease.
D A diastolic murmur.
E Tachycardia up to a heart rate of 100/min improves haemodynamics.

392 A **True**
     B **False**   Surgery should be undertaken after metabolic
                    correction with fluids.
     C **True**
     D **False**   It is hypokalaemic, hypochloraemic alkalosis.
     E **True**

393 A **True**   Ventricular hypertrophy increases the oxygen
                    demand and raised end-diastolic pressure reduces
                    coronary blood flow.
     B **True**   This is due to the thick and poorly compliant
                    myocardium.
     C **True**   Because of increased LVEDP.
     D **True**   Diastolic function is affected earlier than systolic.
     E **True**

394 A **True**
     B **True**
     C **False**   PCWP will be increased as well.
     D **False**   Inotropic response to β agonists is reduced.
     E **True**   Pulmonary congestion leads to increased total lung
                    water.

395 A **True**
     B **True**
     C **True**
     D **False**   Systemic vascular resistance, if altered at all, is
                    increased.
     E **False**   A β-blocker may mask the clinical signs of
                    hypoglycaemia; it does not cause a rise in blood
                    sugar on its own.

396 A **True**
     B **True**
     C **True**   This is due to narrowing of the ostia or to increased
                    myocardial oxygen demand.
     D **False**   A systolic murmur is characteristic.
     E **False**   Tachycardia is poorly tolerated as it reduces time for
                    diastolic filling.

397 Hepatorenal syndrome in a patient with cirrhosis is usually associated with:

A Raised serum creatinine with polyurea.
B Good prognosis following treatment with dopamine.
C Intense vasoconstriction of the afferent arterioles.
D Tubular debris producing high intraluminal pressure.
E Marked improvement on normalisation of liver function.

398 A transplanted heart:

A Does not respond to atropine.
B Is unable to increase heart rate during hypovolaemia.
C Has downregulation of the β receptors.
D Does not respond to catecholamines.
E Beats at a rate of 90–100 beats/min.

399 Indications for preoperative dialysis in a patient with renal failure include:

A Pericardial tamponade.
B Platelet dysfunction with increased bleeding.
C Congestive heart failure.
D Hypervolaemia.
E Uraemic symptoms.

400 The relationship between $PaCO_2$ (x-axis) and ventilatory minute volume (y-axis) becomes steeper with:

A Hypoxia.
B Narcotics.
C Chronic obstructive pulmonary disease.
D Anaemia.
E Central sleep apnoea.

397 A **False**   Oliguria is common.
     B **False**   This syndrome heralds a bad prognosis and, unlike
                     acute tubular necrosis, does not show a good
                     response to dopamine, diuretics or ACE inhibitors.
     C **True**
     D **False**   This is a feature of acute tubular necrosis.
     E **True**

398 A **True**   As it does not have a vagal supply.
     B **True**
     C **False**   These receptors are upregulated.
     D **False**   It responds promptly to exogenous catecholamines.
     E **True**

399 A **True**
     B **True**
     C **True**
     D **True**
     E **True**
     Other indications are metabolic acidosis and hyperkalaemia.

400 A **True**   Hypoxia sensitises the ventilatory response to   ˜
                     carbon dioxide.
     B **False**   Narcotics depress the response.
     C **False**   COPD depresses the response.
     D **True**   Due to the relative hypoxia.
     E **False**   The problem here is a lack of ventilatory response to
                     carbon dioxide.

Subject index

Appropriate question numbers are given

ANAESTHESIA FOR CARDIAC AND THORACIC SURGERY

34, 35, 36, 46, 62, 74, 75, 80, 84,
92, 95, 114, 115, 124, 131, 135,
154, 155, 156, 157, 161, 175, 177,
193, 194, 195, 196, 201, 202, 211,
219, 222, 233, 234, 235, 237, 241,
242, 251, 273, 274, 275, 276, 282,
297, 300, 313, 322, 333, 353, 354,
356, 393, 394

ANAESTHESIA FOR NEUROSURGERY

30, 31, 37, 57, 71, 77, 109, 136, 138,
149, 150, 173, 189, 190, 208, 229,
230, 246, 269, 270, 286, 309, 310,
326, 335, 341, 349, 350, 390

ANAESTHESIA IN PATIENTS WITH ORGAN FAILURE INCLUDING THOSE FOR TRANSPLANT SURGERY

39, 40, 78, 79, 83, 86, 87, 118, 119,
120, 158, 159, 163, 213, 238, 239,
254, 278, 279, 295, 318, 319, 323,
330, 334, 336, 357, 358, 359, 397,
398, 399

ANAESTHESIA FOR PAEDIATRIC SURGERY

32, 33, 72, 73, 85, 102, 111, 112,
113, 151, 152, 153, 191, 192, 231,
232, 267, 271, 272, 311, 312, 351,
352, 385, 391, 392

CONDUCT OF ANAESTHESIA

10, 11, 13, 26, 49, 50, 51, 56, 58,
59, 67, 72, 76, 89, 90, 97, 98, 99,
116, 117, 121, 129, 130, 137, 140,
146, 154, 156, 157, 167, 168, 169,
171, 177, 185, 196, 210, 211, 235,
236, 237, 238, 242, 249, 250, 261,
262, 275, 276, 283, 289, 290, 301,
305, 316, 341, 347, 350, 358, 372,
373, 376, 377

MEDICINE

1, 2, 3, 14, 22, 35, 38, 40, 43, 44,
45, 46, 61, 62, 66, 76, 78, 83, 91,
118, 121, 123, 124, 132, 135, 156,
160, 163, 164, 171, 174, 194, 195,
201, 202, 203, 204, 211, 233, 235,
236, 237, 241, 243, 251, 276, 277,
278, 281, 282, 283, 288, 289, 294,
295, 298, 315, 316, 319, 320, 321,
322, 323, 329, 331, 333, 354, 355,
357, 361, 362, 363, 364, 370, 374,
396

PAIN MANAGEMENT AND REGIONAL ANALGESIA (INCLUDING ANATOMY)

23, 24, 50, 55, 63, 64, 103, 104,
107, 141, 143, 144, 147, 153, 178,
180, 183, 184, 187, 209, 217, 223,
224, 226, 227, 257, 263, 264, 297,
299, 303, 304, 306, 343, 344, 346,
358, 383, 386

PHARMACOLOGY

1, 4, 5, 8, 9, 10, 17, 18, 22, 26, 41,
44, 45, 48, 49, 54, 65, 72, 75, 80,

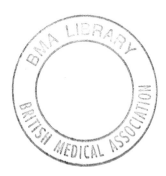